HOW TO EAT LIKE A *Normal* PERSON

HOW TO EAT LIKE A Normal PERSON

KAIT RICHARDSON, RDN, LD

Accomplishing
Innovation Press

Dedication

To my beautiful mother and role model Ericka, my colleague Megan Poczekaj who gave me a place to practice my passion, and the women who inspired this book. Thank you for trusting in me.

Table of Contents

Disclaimer

Kait is a Registered Dietitian, not a licensed therapist or medical doctor. This information is for educational and entertainment purposes only. It is not meant to be a substitute for mental health counseling or medical advice.

Testimonials

"I can honestly say that Kait has changed my life for the better. I have gained a completely new perspective on what it means for me to live a healthy lifestyle in a nonjudgemental & warm environment. The tools I have learned through my sessions with Kait have been sustainable and have improved my overall well-being physically and mentally. You can tell that Kait genuinely cares about her clients and their success. I cannot recommend Kait enough - worth every penny!"

-Katie Love, Real Life Client

"Kait is super knowledgeable and kind... literally the epitome of professionalism and kindness. I felt no shame at all and left [our appointment] feeling inspired to make a few manageable yet key lifestyle changes. Truly feel like I've found what will work for me while being sustainable. There are no fads here, only real nutrition science."

-Caitlin Rohm, Real Life Client

After about 3 years of yo-yo dieting, I pretty much came to the realization that I need professional help. Mostly, to learn how to eat a balanced, nutritious "diet" that I can sustain long term because even though some diets gave results, they aren't maintainable (as I've learned the hard way- to a high cost). My opinion and first impression [of] Kait is that she is very much aware of the modern struggles that we all face- the conflicting information out there, social media, etc. The unhealthy patterns we set. She listens very well and is able to get to the root of the problems immediately. It feels like she really knows her craft and has mastered her job... I would recommend to anyone!"

- Jolyne Gaudet, Real Life Client

"As a former yo-yo dieter and a licensed psychologist, I can say with full confidence that Kait's methods are the real deal. Even as a mental health professional with experience treating eating disorders, I struggled to break free from fear and anxiety about weight gain, and all-or-nothing thinking related to food. I reached out to Kait after some very stressful life experiences and weight gain that left me feeling like I "failed." I found myself stuck between two worlds— one that normalized restrictive dieting at all costs, and one that was staunchly anti-dieting (for good reason). Kait helped me create my own definition of health, reconnect with my values, and gain trust in myself so I no longer worry about "falling off the wagon." I know when life happens I can just pick up where I left off. Yes, I lost weight, but far more importantly, I gained a new mindset and deeper love for myself."

-Samantha Sciarrillo, PsyD & Real Life Client

"As a woman who has battled disordered eating for virtually my entire life, I was in very real need of a nutritionist who could understand the path my life's journey took me on, and provide guidance on how to correct behaviors that had become ingrained within me. Kait Richardson's knowledge, caring and ability to identify with me on a personal level gave me the confidence to go outside my comfort zone and make the necessary changes in my dietary habits that put me on a new path toward happiness and a healthy relationship with food. Without Kait, I would, without a doubt, be on my 35th year of disordered eating with no end in sight. I highly recommend Kait Richardson for anyone needing nutritional advice on every level."

-Kristin Green, Real Life Client

"Meeting Kait has been an absolute blessing in my life. She has helped me work through multiple food issues I had and finally got me to break the cycle of yo-yo dieting and other unhealthy eating habits. Over time I noticed my weight steadily drop and my overall health improve. Kait is also very culturally sensitive. I'm Hispanic and Asian, so in the past I've encountered "nutritionists" that would discount the foods from my culture and insist I eat foods that I didn't enjoy. Kait was able to coach me in how I could still eat healthy and enjoy the food I grew up with. Kait is not about crash diets or fad diets, she helped me develop a whole new healthy lifestyle. I did six months of coaching and two rounds of The Daily Accountability Program, and it was absolutely worth it for the permanent changes I now see in my life."

- Karen Anthony, Real Life Client

"For me, the journey of maintaining healthy often becomes so over-whelming and gets put on the back burner (especially during the holidays: Thanksgiving, Christmas and New Years). That's why I researched and decided to obtain Kait's services. Investing in Kait was the best decision I could have made for my health. Kait educated me on what to look at in foods, to add more fruits and vegetables in my meals and I no longer have the sweet tooth I once had (and honestly, I never thought I would live without). I lost weight, sleep better, and feel more energetic than ever! I also love and appreciate her podcasts with Kait's partner Megan. Thank you guys for doing what you do and how convenient you do it!"

-Jeannie Maeztu, Real Life Client

None of these clients or their stories were referenced in this book. To learn how to work with Kait, visit www.kaitrichardsonrd.com.

Part 1

Normal Eaters

This is **not** a diet book. You will not be given tips and tricks on how to lose weight quickly, nor will I recommend "super" foods for fat loss because frankly, there is no such thing. This book will not shame you for enjoying a frosted cupcake at your niece's birthday party or make you question whether carrots are "bad" (they aren't), because they have too much sugar (they don't). There will be no weighing every gram of rice, fasting until noon, or forcing down chalky protein shakes for the sake of weight loss. Why? Because this is a health book written to teach you how to *eat like a normal person*, and restrictive dieting is anything but normal.

Since Normal Eaters are never "on" a diet, they're never "off" one either. This means they're not restricting themselves to only steamed broccoli and baked tofu all week just to stuff their face with spicy chicken tenders and onion rings all weekend. They don't have to earn "cheat meals" because that term doesn't exist in a Normal Eater's vocabulary!

Normal Eaters are not obsessed over the calories in a meal, nor are they concerned about whether a food is "good" or "bad." They don't feel morally superior when they order a spinach salad at lunch, nor do they experience guilt after eating a burger with a bun instead of a soggy lettuce wrap.

1

After a stressful or emotional day, Normal Eaters don't unwind with an entire box of graham crackers or bottle of wine. If they indulge in cravings, Normal Eaters don't berate themselves for not having enough "willpower" or "discipline." They don't punish themselves the next day with extra cardio or bland egg white omelets.

They're human after all, and enjoying a treat in the context of a balanced diet doesn't make them a failure.

Exercise is about more than just weight loss to Normal Eaters, so they fuel well before a tough workout instead of staving off hunger with a measly rice cake. They don't skip meals in an effort to save calories for the evening meal. Instead, they give their body food when they're hungry and stop when they are comfortably full.

If Normal Eaters decide to lose weight, they don't restrict their daily calories to 1200 or less because they know they'll end up binging on sugar and grease all weekend. Instead, they become more mindful around food. Normal Eaters focus on fueling their bodies with as many nutritious foods as possible without restricting sweets and snacks. The few that bother with weighing themselves do not let daily fluctuations on the scale dictate how they feel about themselves. They focus on changing their lifestyle, so they don't lose the same 5 to 15 pounds over and over again.

Most importantly, Normal Eaters accept and love their body. Instead of constantly depriving it or overworking it, they honor their basic human needs for food and rest.

Seem out of reach? I assure you, it's not! No matter how many crazy diets you've tried (or how many you've given up on), it's 100% possible to learn how to eat like a normal person. You **can** gain control of food without having to restrict yourself. It's going to take some rewiring, but we can get there.

Death to Diets

If I were queen of the world, I'd outlaw fad diets, fat loss pills, and bogus meal plans. Anyone who defies my orders would be punished by having a taste of their own restrictive eating medicine for life. No more croissants with butter, no more coffee with cream, only Americanos and ground turkey with spinach for the rest of eternity! Personally, I'd take a prison cell before I'd give up my oat milk lattes.

Alas, I'm not a diet dictator who can enforce rules on diet culture, but I am a registered dietitian. Therefore, I've made it my life's purpose to share how diets are not only harmful but get in the way of achieving long-term health.

Learning how to eat like a Normal Person can help you improve your relationship to food and maintain sustainable results. It resolves the patterns than keep women stuck, including the following:

- Yo-yo dieting

- Obsessive calorie, macronutrient, or food tracking

- Anxiety about "good" and "bad" foods

- Confusion over how and when to eat

- Emotional eating

- Binge eating

- Orthorexia[1]

- Distrust of oneself around food

Not only are these struggles mentally and physically exhausting, they are extremely isolating. Sure, many women admit they'd like to lose weight or eat less sugar, but how many will come out and admit to scarfing down an entire box of cereal after ordering the garden salad at lunch?

Because of social media and the pressure to appear flawless, not enough of women are vulnerable enough to talk about how deeply they struggle with eating and body image. Consequently, women of all shapes, sizes, and backgrounds suffer in silence. When too few women admit how they're eating behind closed doors, it may cause you to question what is wrong with *you*. You may think, *How come everyone else has it all together with food while I can't control myself around a bag of stale gummy worms? Why can't I just eat like a normal freakin' person?*

---

[1] *Orthorexia is an obsession with healthy eating with associated restrictive behaviors*

As a registered dietitian who has the privilege to help women with similar concerns, I want to assure you that you are far from alone. There is **nothing** wrong with you. No matter how messy you think your relationship with food is, someone else has been through your pain and come out the other side stronger. And even more women, regardless of their waist circumference and cultural upbringing, have overcome their unwanted eating habits and transformed their lives using the techniques outlined in this book.

You are 100% capable of the same.

Why We Struggle

Over the years, I have seen a steady rise in the number of clients whose primary goal is to improve their relationship with food. More women are becoming self-aware of their disordered behaviors around food and are seeking help. After trying out every fad diet in the sun, they want to find a balanced approach that works.

I've heard countless stories from women who went on their first diet in middle school, or whose mothers would sign them up for weight loss programs when they hit puberty and their bodies naturally changed. I once had a client whose mother thought she was being helpful when she packed her diet shakes for breakfast and scolded her for wanting grapes because they had "too much sugar." Little did her mom know, rules around food planted the seed for years of body image issues and disordered eating. This is also the case for women who grew up with caregivers who dieted, spoke negatively about their own body, or upheld strict standards about how a woman's figure should look.

Beauty standards vary from culture to culture. My Latina clients often tell me, "I'm either too skinny or too fat. My grandmother will tell me I've gained weight, then get offended when I don't ask for a second helping."

Asian American women share stories of how the matriarchs of their family aren't afraid to tell them they look fat in a photo or point out weight gain in front of others. Culture or not, it's hurtful.

How women feel about their body doesn't stop outside the home. Social media influencers and so-called "medical gurus" promoting supplements and quick fixes also cause lasting harm to women's mental and metabolic health. Even well-meaning medical professionals pre-scribing diet pills or low-carb diets intensify feelings of confusion and stress over what to eat. When the diet inevitably fails, the woman blames herself instead of the approach. After all, if a doctor or "health coach" swears by a certain protocol, it must be right...

Right? If only! There is no one-size-fits-all approach, which is why women must stop listening to arbitrary diet advice and practice listening to their own bodies.

We, as women, are becoming farther removed from the intuitive knowledge about which foods feel best for our bodies. Instead of reflecting on our own experiences around food, society instructs us to Google the answer from external sources. Dieting teaches us we cannot trust our intuition because an "expert" told us we were wrong. When we lose our ability to regulate hunger and satiety cues, it leads to disordered eating, confusion, and guilt.

Never mind the intense hunger pains you feel at 10 AM if you're not allowed to break your fast until noon! By suppressing your need for food with hot lemon water or black coffee, you're teaching your brain that your needs don't matter. You are training yourself to value the opinions and ideas of others more than your own. **In the age of self-love and self-care, dieting is the ultimate form of self-betrayal.**

We suffer through seasons of rule-following with the hopes we'll transform and finally feel happy. We buy the lies diet culture feeds us without realizing, when we follow statutes created & marketed by someone else, we're only deepening feelings of self-rejection and distrust.

We continue to fall prey to the siren call of diet programs and quick fixes not because we're dumb or naive. We do it because believing we're on the right path feels comforting, like we've finally found the magic pill that will solve our discomfort. "Proven Methods" and cook-ie-cutter meal plans trick us into thinking we'll find evergreen hap-piness and body confidence on the other side of 10, 20, or 50 lbs. Starting a diet is not a solution; it's a temporary distraction from feeling unhappy with your body image, health, or lifestyle.

Even if weight is shed during a diet, it rarely lasts. Diets don't teach you how to eat for life. They teach you to restrict until you inevitably can't. For most of us, we can only reject the messages from our body and blindly follow a diet for so long.

Diet Addiction

Why aren't there more role models are out there sharing how to eat like a healthy, normal person? Well, compared to an extreme approach like the ketogenic diet or raw veganism, practical advice isn't sexy! A healthy lifestyle takes time and patience. It can't be packaged and marketed to offer immediate fat loss.

For example, pretend you're following a notorious 1200 calorie diet. After a week of drastically undereating, you lose three pounds. You know the loss is from water weight or you pooped before you stepped on the scale, but your brain lights up and you think, *It's working! Hallelujah, it's really working!* Then you eat fried chicken and syrupy waffles at your best friend's birthday brunch, just to regain the three pounds you lost. Panic sets in but restricting food after a setback feels harder than before. To make yourself feel better about giving up, you promise to start over on Monday.

On days when we are dissatisfied with our body image, our brains remember short-lived victories. Desperate to feel better, we vow to cut carbs or track calories again because our brains learned restriction leads to quick results. An unsustainable behavior was reinforced. **This is why dieting feels addictive,** no matter how many times you regain the weight or fall off track.

For some, diets end gradually. A stolen French fry off a friend's plate, half a donut at the office on a Friday, or an extra pump of vanilla syrup in an almond milk latte- each bend of the rules adds up. At the breaking point, they say *screw it* and order the truffle mac n' cheese at dinner. For others, diets come to a screeching halt when a vacation to the Bahamas or an innocent "cheat" weekend blows them off course entirely. After the fun of overindulging is over, these dieters find themselves back at square one (and square one is *not* a fun place to be when you start from a place of self-hatred or disgust).

No matter how it ends, dieters find themselves diving head first into a new diet a few weeks or months later, forgetting all the pain and hardship they endured from the previous attempt. Their desperation to lose weight fast keeps them fighting a never-ending war against their bodies.

The kicker? Your body always wins.

But the good news is you are your body.
Fueling it well means you win, too.

You Are Your Body

After forming relationships and engaging in thousands of hours of deep conversations with clients, I noticed there are patterns among women who float between diets, can't sustain results, and feel disconnected from their bodies.

One major theme is that they fret over the small stuff, like if it's OK to use one tablespoon of almond milk creamer in their coffee or eat fruit after 2:30 p.m. They ask me if it's best to drink lemon water at room temperature and are concerned about the sugar content of carrots. Instead of focusing on the big picture, they hyper-fixate on irrelevant, microscopic details.

Nine times out of ten, these women have tried restrictive approaches, such as:

- Ketogenic diets (more about this on page 21)

- Intermittent fasting

- Macronutrient counting

- Low-carb eating

- Going gluten or dairy free[2]

- Plant-based eating[3]

- Group weight loss programs

- 1200 calorie diets

- Juice cleanses and detoxes

- Fat burner pills

---

[2] *There is nothing wrong with ditching gluten or dairy, if it suits your preferences or medical needs. If the sole purpose is weight loss, and it results in overeating these foods later, it's not helpful.*

[3] *The above statement also applies to veganism or vegetarianism.*

- Clean eating

These diets are all the same lump of coal wrapped in different, well-marketed packages. Not only do they demonize certain foods or restrict portions, they conflict with one another. It's confusing when one diet is telling followers to eat every six hours while another says to eat only once!

Women who ping-pong between diets begin to believe they can only see results if the process is strenuous. They dive headfirst into the shallow waters of 60 day sugar detoxes and lengthy diets such as Whole30 thinking that hard equals change. I beg to differ. When pushing too hard leads to burnout, any meaningful change doesn't stick. The entire process was a waste of time and energy.

Diets and extreme workout challenges also trick women into believing anything less than 100% effort is a waste. If they're not drenched in sweat after a 60-minute workout, why bother with a lower impact 20-minute one? If they eat more than their allotted number of carbohydrates in a day, why stop there? Might as well keep going and start over tomorrow, right?

No! That's not how *normal people eat*.

Women with this mindset are stuck spinning their wheels, wondering why the hell they can't control themselves around food. The mere thought of eating without following a plan stresses them out because they don't trust themselves not to finish a sleeve of crackers in one sitting or order a large lemonade with lunch. So they sign up for weight loss program after weight loss program, which paradoxically worsens their relationship to food.

If you ask them what eating healthy means, they can't tell you.

Ironically, they fear "bad" foods but overeat them.

They lose weight just to regain it.

Archetypally, they are All-or-Nothing Dieters.

The All-Or-Nothing Dieter Archetype

In the chapters of this book, you'll hear the stories of six different women who embody the **All-Or-Nothing Dieter Archetype**.

An **archetype** is a broad term used to define a pattern of behavior. For example, the archetype of a Caregiver can be described as loving, compassionate, and nurturing. Caregivers are maternal in nature and prioritize helping others. Mother Teresa embodies The Caregiver archetype.

Archetypes have sub-archetypes. Sub-archetypes are equal to main archetypes, but they have characteristics that differentiate them from the main archetype. Examples of The Caregiver sub-archetype include The Guardian and The Samaritan[4]. Both are compassionate in nature, but the Guardian is marked by her need to protect and The Samaritan her need to relieve suffering.

To give a quick example, the **All-Or-Nothing Dieter** bounces from one extreme program to the next while measuring her self-worth based on outcomes. This is why she is drawn to diets: she has a clear goal, and she is motivated to follow step-by-step processes to do so, no matter how difficult or strict the plan. If she follows the plan perfectly, then she deems herself worthy. As soon as she slips up, she falls apart. One day she's tracking every bite in a weight loss app, the next she's pretending donuts don't have calories. She works out every day for a week just to skip the gym entirely the following month. She's eating a "clean" lunch but grabbing egg rolls and fried rice for dinner.

Within the **All-Or-Nothing Dieter Archetype**, I have identified sub-archetypes. The six sub-archetypes discussed in the chapters of this book are:

- **The Food Tracker**

- **The Perfectionist**

- **The Emotional Eater**

- **The Yo-Yo Dieter**

- **The Binge Eater**

- **The Cardio Bunny**

It is possible to embody the characteristics of more than one sub-archetype or a few elements of each. To determine which sub-archetype(s) you identify with, you must understand the **shadow tendencies** of each.

---

[4] *This concept is explained in the book Archetypes in Branding: A Toolkit for Creatives and Strategists by Margaret Hartwell (Author), Joshua C. Chen (Author)*

Integrating the Shadow Side

Every sub-archetype has a **shadow,** a term coined by Swiss psychoanalyst Carl Jung to describe the elements of personality that do not align with who we want to be. Our **shadow tendencies** are often buried in our unconscious mind and consist of our weaknesses and repressed ideas, making it uncomfortable to examine this side of our personality! After all, few of us want to admit our faults.

The overarching shadow of The Caregiver Archetype is self-sacrifice to help others. Constantly putting the needs of her friends, family, and colleagues before her own may cause her to build resentment, ultimately harming her relationships and personal wellbeing. However, the self-aware Caregiver can identify her people-pleasing pattern and create boundaries when appropriate. This way, she remains true to her helpful nature without giving up her own needs.

The overarching shadow of All-or-Nothing Dieters is restrictive eating and extremism with food or body image. One of **The Emotional Eater's** shadows is using food to cope with stress or sadness, while **The Yo-Yo Dieter** starts extreme dieting to temporarily ease her anxiety and discontent with her body. As you'll learn through this book, any shadow can be managed with self-awareness and effort to evolve.

Jung believed many people deny their shadow side and project it onto others. This may explain why a woman with insecurities about her figure is vocal about the physical imperfections of others instead of working on her own self-acceptance. She may be in denial with how deeply insecure she is, because she has not taken the time to examine her shadow side. Until she faces these hidden insecurities and thought patterns, she'll continue to criticize and deflect negativity about herself onto other women.

Although it can be uncomfortable, it's critical to face our unhealthy thoughts and patterns around food and body image head on. Bringing our shadow into the light allows us to blossom into the healthiest version of ourselves.

The beginning of each chapter lists common shadow tendencies of each sub-archetype. Reading each chapter can help you identify, understand, and resolve root causes of shadow tendencies. You may find you align with the shadow tendencies of **The Binge Eater** while also embodying characteristics of **The Perfectionist** in specific situations or environments.

While both **The Binge Eater** and **The Perfectionist** go from one extreme to the next, the root cause of the **The Binge Eater's** issues with food stem from self-rejection while **The Perfectionist's** issues come from a fear of disapproval from others. This means they will have to incorporate different techniques to help them find peace with food.

Once **The Food Tracker** realizes counting every calorie or weighing every gram of rice actually leaves her feeling more out of control with food, she can focus on the big picture of how and what she's eating. From there, she can feel relaxed around food while creating structure by meal planning and monitoring her energy, workouts, and mood. Now she's in control of food instead of food controlling her!

When **The Cardio Bunny** understands her fear of gaining weight if she eats carbohydrates is sabotaging her fitness goals, she can strategically integrate the right fuel to improve her performance. By using food as a tool, she'll feel better, without worrying about gaining weight.

It's critical to note your goal should not be to judge yourself for possessing specific shadow tendencies. Shadows give us depth! Having deep-rooted fears and struggles is all part of the human experience, and your mission is to recognize your shadow tendencies and integrate them in a healthy, proactive way. One-size-fits-all diets won't help everyone—we all have different shadow sides!

Regardless of which sub-archetypes you most closely align with, I recommend reading through them in order. You'll learn eating strategies and mindset shifts from each chapter that will help you address your shadow tendencies and become the healthiest version of you. **Each chapter will share the following:**

1. The shadow tendencies of each sub-archetype

2. The story inspired by a client who embodied these shadow tendencies and how they impacted her wellbeing

3. Teach you the strategies I used with each client to help her integrate her shadow side in a healthy way so that she could attain her goals

My mission is to empower you so you can identify what's really at the core of your all-or-nothing dieting struggles, access the mindset tools to overcome them, and utilize evidence-based nutrition strategies to improve your eating habits for good.

As you read each story, you'll come across subsections titled **Your Turn.** Here, you'll be prompted to pause, journal, and incorporate healthy eating strategies into your own life. To help make sense of the recommendations in each chapter, I've provided free resources and recipes at www.kaitrichardsonrd.com.

Ready to stop starving and suffering to lose weight? Then let's get into it! After all, you can't live a full life on an empty stomach.

Fundamentals of Balanced Nutrition

Evidence-based information is fundamental to improving your relationship to food and reaching your individual goals, but to apply the lessons from this book, you need a basic understanding of nutrition.

Every client mentioned received the following education before they set individual goals. Many of the strategies are most effective if you understand these concepts, so I suggest revisiting this chapter as often as you need!

Food is Energy

Your body requires energy in the form of **calories** to function. Calories (energy) come from food, not vitamins, pills, or caffeine. Although you may feel a jolt after drinking an iced coffee or energy drink, neither provides you with actual *fuel* from calories and they should **not** be substitutes for real food.

It's easy to think about how activities such as working out burn calories, but we forget basic life-sustaining functions, such as your heart pumping, also require energy. Other functions that require calories include:

- Breathing

- Speaking

- Thinking

- Digestion

- Menstruation

- Cleaning

- Walking/Exercising

- Repairing cuts/bruises or skin tears

- Rebuilding muscle fibers after a workout

The bare minimum amount of total energy it requires to keep you alive is known as your *Basal Metabolic Rate* (BMR). Imagine you were lying in bed all day and not moving a finger. The amount of energy you would burn doing absolutely nothing is your BMR.

Everyone's BMR is different, and it changes throughout your life. Your BMR depends on a variety of factors: age, biological sex, weight, muscle mass, body fat percentage, activity levels, genetics, etc. Though not required, you can test your BMR at analysis sites offering Dexa Scans or InBody machines. There are predictive equations[5] online, but take these with a grain of salt. Estimates cannot account for factors such as genetics or diet history. Rarely (and I mean, *rarely)* do I see women under the age of 60 with BMRs less than 1200, so do not I recommend most women in that age group eat less than 1200 calories per day without a BMR test.

"But Kait, my 1200 calorie diet worked for me 5 years ago."

If you regained the weight and/or have a miserable relationship to food, no, it did not. Quick fixes and starvation diets don't work because your body's #1 priority is to keep you alive, not to fit into last

---

[5] *Mifflin St. Jeor is a common equation used to calculate basal metabolic rates.*

year's jeans. When your brain senses it's not receiving enough energy to function, it intrinsically encourages you to eat and therefore, live. One way your brain does this is by secreting hunger hormones, which makes you want to eat *more* than usual. You may also find yourself having frequent thoughts about eating or struggle to find the energy to exercise or play. Can you see how this is a recipe for weight regain?

In response to an extreme caloric restriction, biology *always* wins by sending dieters intense signals to eat or rest. The will to live is incredible, but if you've been battling your weight for years, it can feel incredibly frustrating.

All-or-Nothing Dieters misplace this frustration in one of two ways. They give up on their goals entirely, or they push their limits harder, desperate to burn fat fast. When they could be slowing down to work *with* their bodies, they work tirelessly against them by restricting more food.

Instead of blaming biology, All-or-Nothing Dieters believe they lack willpower or motivation. Yet these are some of the most accomplished, achievement-oriented individuals I've ever met. To claim they are unmotivated is a lie they're telling themselves to make sense of their poor eating habits. Truth is, even the most disciplined person will have trouble staying consistent when they're not fueling properly. The BNT Protocol fixes that.

The BNT Protocol

When it comes to fueling the body, I teach my clients to follow **The BNT Protocol.** BNT stands for:

1. **Balanced** meals and snacks

2. **Nutritious** foods 80% of the time

3. **Timing** for fuel every 3-6 hours

How to Balance Meals & Snacks:

Food contains three macronutrients: protein, fat, and carbohydrate, and all provide calories for your body to utilize in different ways.

Protein aids in body tissue growth, structure, and repair. This includes not only your muscles but your hair, skin, and nail strength!

Protein also keeps you fuller longer, so you're not as hungry between meals. For those who like numbers and totals, aim to eat 0.8-1 grams of protein per pound of your ideal weight most days (i.e, if you're 150 pounds, eat at least 120 grams).

Does this seem like a lot? Not if you break it down into 20-50 grams of protein at each meal and at least 10 grams of snacks.[6] Spacing your protein intake throughout the day will help with satiety and muscle protein synthesis, a fancy term for the process of building muscle tissue.

Dietary Fat provides slow, sustained energy, and will also keep you satisfied between meals. It insulates your organs and provides the building blocks for hormones. Fat does not make you fat—you need it to survive!

Carbohydrates break down in the body as *glucose,* which is your body's preferred source of energy. This means it will readily use carbs to fuel your body. As you'll learn throughout this book, consuming enough carbohydrates throughout the day will help you have more control over food.

Because carbohydrate and fat needs vary widely per individual, I do not give general recommendations for total carbohydrate and fat intake.

Eating a balance of macronutrients is crucial for **blood sugar control**. You can think of your blood sugar as the barometer for your energy, cravings, appetite, and mood. Carbohydrates increase blood sugar while dietary fats do not. Protein has a slight impact on blood sugar. When you don't have enough carbohydrates, or *glucose*, your blood sugar will drop over time.

Symptoms of low blood sugar include fatigue, irritability, and cravings for sugar. When your blood sugar has dropped too low, your body is desperate for large servings of quick energy to keep you alive. No matter how much you want to eat healthy or follow a low-calorie diet, biology will drive you to eat refined carbohydrates like chips or candy in excess. Low-carb dieters who only eat protein and vegetables (like Aniyah, The Cardio Bunny), or meal-skippers (like Sarah, The Emotional Eater) experience massive cravings in the afternoon and evenings for this reason.

On the flip side, eating too many carbohydrates and not enough protein or dietary fat during the day will cause a quick spike in blood

---

[6] *Please don't stress if your snack bar contains 9 grams instead of 10 grams. These are recommendations, not laws.*

sugar. This is especially true when the carbohydrate is ultra-processed, refined, or high in sugar. You'll feel a quick jolt of energy followed by a blood sugar crash, leading to more cravings for sugar. People who experience this roller coaster of blood sugar spikes may feel like sugar addicts, but as soon as they begin balancing their nutrients, they feel more in control over their appetite and cravings. Managing your blood sugar is the only way you'll be able to sustainably reach your health and weight goals without feeling miserable.

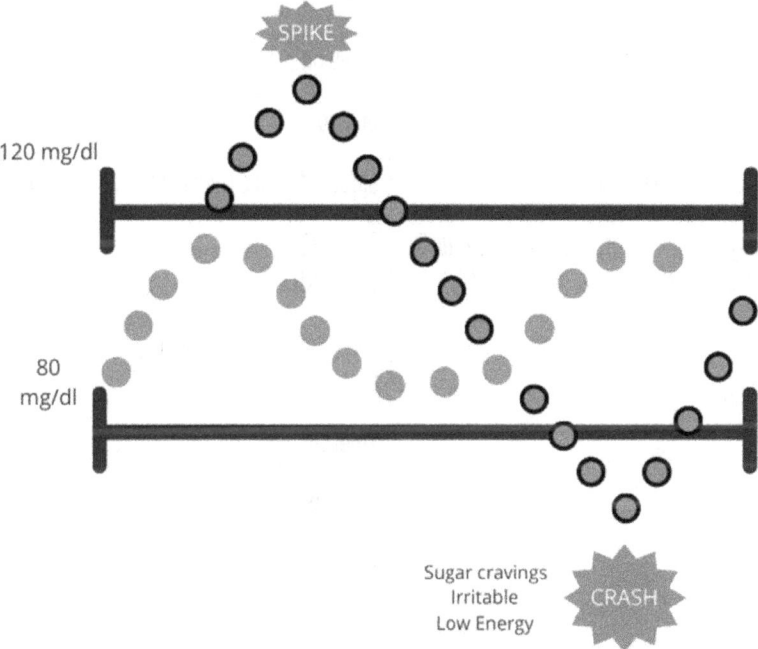

⬤ blood sugar effects from a high carb meal

⬤ blood sugar effects after balanced, whole food meal

SPIKE

120 mg/dl

80 mg/dl

Sugar cravings
Irritable
Low Energy

CRASH

What if you're in a situation where eating a balanced meal or snack isn't possible, or you're not hungry enough for anything more than a pear? Don't sweat it! As long as the vast majority of your meals contain a combination of complex carbs, protein, and healthy fats, eating a boiled egg without a carb or buttered toast without protein won't make or break you.

If you're overwhelmed or confused, don't worry! Throughout this book, there will be plenty of examples of balanced vs. unbalanced meals to help you nail this concept.

Eating Nutritious Foods 80% of the Time

Not all carbs, proteins, and fats are created equal.

Nutritious carbohydrates contain fiber, vitamins, minerals, and phytonutrients. The best sources have less than 3 grams of *added sugar* per serving. The table below lists examples of complex carbohydrates.

Healthy Sources of Carbohydrates

Beans (any!)	Milk
Berries	Pumpkin
Brown rice	Quinoa
Chickpeas or chickpea pasta	Sprouted grains (bread, tortillas, and crackers)
Greek yogurt (look for brands with *less than* 3 grams of **added** sugar)	Squash (acorn, butternut, or spaghetti squash)
Hummus	Starchy vegetables (beets, carrots, peas)
Fruit (any!)	Steel cut or old fashioned oats
Lentils	Sweet potatoes
	Whole grains (barley, farro, couscous)

Table 1.2.1

Non-starchy vegetables such as broccoli, zucchini, cauliflower, and bell peppers contain small amounts of carbohydrates. They should be included in most meals but **not** as a substitute for the carbs listed above.

Forget what you've heard about fruit being too high in sugar! As long as you pair it with protein, enjoy any and all the fruit you'd like.

Check the nutrition label of protein bars and drinks as they often contain carbohydrates and added sugar.

Oat milk is not listed because unlike rolled or old-fashioned oats, oat milk does not contain fiber. Since there is also no protein or fat present, oat milk is more likely to spike your blood sugar. If you love it, enjoy it alongside a meal with protein and fiber! For those looking for a dairy-free milk with more nutrition, try unsweetened soy milk, hemp seed milk, or coconut milk.

Nutritious Proteins are minimally processed and contain b-vitamins, iron, and minerals like calcium and zinc. The table below lists sources of quality protein.

Healthy Sources of Protein

Animal Sources:	Plant-Based Sources:
Cheese	Beans
Milk	Hemp seeds or hemp seed milk
Fish and shellfish	Edamame
Full-fat cottage cheese	Natural or freshly ground nut butters
Full-fat Greek yogurt	Nuts and seeds (any!)
Grass fed meats	Nut milks fortified with protein
Liver and other organ meats	Plant-based protein bars
Pasture-raised eggs	Plant-based protein powders and shakes made with brown rice, soy, or peas
Poultry (chicken, turkey, duck)	Seeds (hemp, chia, pumpkin)
Protein bars (using whey)	Soy: Tempeh, tofu
Protein shakes	Soy milk

Table 1.2.2

Animal proteins contain all 20 of the essential amino acids and with the exception of soy, are more readily absorbed than plant-based proteins. Vegans and vegetarians must ensure they're eating a variety of non-animal protein sources to meet their needs. Supplements such as protein shakes and bars can be helpful! Be sure to check food labels— plant-based meat alternatives are not always nutritionally equivalent to the animal source. Certain vegan burgers have less protein than a turkey burger, so additional protein may be needed in that meal.

Nutritious Fats promote heart health and lower cholesterol while keeping you full and satisfied. The table below lists sources of healthy fats.

Healthy Sources of Dietary Fat

Avocados	Ground flaxseed
Avocado oil	Nut milk
Coconut (unsweetened)	Nuts and nut butters
Coconut oil (unrefined)	Olives
Chia seeds	Olive oil
Edamame	Pasture-raised egg yolks
Fatty fish (salmon, tuna, mackerel, herring, trout, black cod, sardines)	Seeds and seed butters
	Soy milk

Table 1.2.3

Some brands of nut milks don't contain any real nutrition. They're okay to drink, but should not be used as substitutes for quality fats. Check the nutrition label and look for at least 8 grams of fat per serving with no added sugars.

Grass-fed meats, grass-fed butter, cheese, milk, coconut oil, and full-fat yogurt contain saturated fats, meaning they should be limited for those concerned about cholesterol or cardiovascular disease. If this is you, work with a Registered Dietitian to learn how to integrate these foods into a heart healthy diet.

When building meals or planning snacks, keep in mind some foods such as milk, nuts, or beans contain more than one macronutrient. Full-fat yogurt can count as a source of protein, carbohydrate, and fat. Depending on how hungry you are, you may or may not need to add any additional food.

Ketosis- A Go or A Big No?

If a diet is not sustainable, don't waste your time trying to make it fit. And unless you don't want to eat out, share meals with friends or family, and don't mind eating a stick of butter as a snack, the ketogenic diet is *not* sustainable.

The goal of the ketogenic diet is to get into *ketosis*, a process in which the body is forced to break down fat into ketones to use for energy because there are not enough carbohydrates. It often takes days to weeks for a person to reach ketosis, requiring at least 70% of her total calories to come from dietary fat and no more than 5-10% of her calories from carbohydrates. This means no healthy foods like quinoa, butternut squash, sweet potato, or fruit, except for *maybe* a tiny serving of berries (depending on the context of what else she ate that day). Even vegetables, which contain carbohydrates, must be closely monitored to keep one in a fat-burning state.

You may think, *I can live without apples and carrots. I'll just eat a bunch of bacon cheeseburgers without the bun.* Nope! Eating too much protein from cheese, nuts, and meat can knock you out of ketosis. In the absence of glucose, the body converts the amino acids from protein into glucose during a process called *gluconeogenesis*. The amount of protein it would take to kick someone out of ketosis varies on the individual, but it can be as little as 30-40 grams of protein per day. This means a smidge too much cheese in your egg yolk omelet can knock you out of ketosis! It's a ridiculous diet that only offers short-term results. Don't do it.

Timing Meals

To prevent frequent spikes and drops in blood sugar, aim to eat a balanced, nutritious meal every 3-6 of your waking hours. Going over 6 hours without fuel may lead to overeating or binge eating. Feeling hungry every 1-2 hours likely means you're under-fueling at meals--eat more protein, dietary **fat, and/or fiber** to stay satiated. If you are grazing every hour out of boredom or stress, create boundaries around how often you eat to stay accountable (more on this in The Perfectionist chapter).

When people tell me they're not hungry in the morning, there are several reasons:

1. They overeat before bed and are still full from the previous night's feast

2. They suppress their appetite with coffee, tea, or energy drinks

3. They're distracted by household tasks, work, or family

Once the day slows down and the caffeine wears off, the body feels ravenous! It's at this point people reach for candy, chips, or convenience foods. To break this cycle, eat within 3 hours of waking most days, **before** or **with** your first coffee.

What about Weight Loss Injections?

Are weight loss injections like semaglutide, tirzeptide, and liraglutide[7] miracle drugs or just another gimmick that will mess with your metabolism? From my discussions with diplomats of the American Board of Obesity Medicine and my growing pool of clients who choose to take semaglutide or tirzepitide, it sounds like it depends on the individual and her usage of the medication.

Weight loss injections are indicated for those with a Body Mass Index (BMI) of over 30 or individuals with a BMI of 27 with a pre-existing medical condition such as type 2 diabetes, high cholesterol,

---

[7] *These are the active ingredients in common medications like Ozempic®, Mounjaro®,* and *Wegovy®.*

hypertension, or insulin resistance. Some folks using the drugs have ugly side effects such as nausea or vomiting while others experience no unwanted symptoms[8].

Working with a trusted medical doctor is crucial, as he or she can appropriately screen your health and determine if a weight loss injection is right for you. Your doctor can also adjust form and dose of anti-obesity medicines to manage side effects and results.

As a registered dietitian, I have major concerns about injections being abused by those with a history of eating disorders and individuals who are not obese or diabetic but want a quick fix to weight loss. Semaglutide was originally used to treat type 2 diabetes and obesity, not help otherwise healthy individuals lose 10 pounds before vacation or quickly shed 12 pounds of excess baby weight.

Why? For one, our country is already experiencing drug shortages. Abusing a weight loss injection means someone who really needs it may not have access. Second, using a weight loss injection to quickly drop weight can read havoc on your metabolism. Studies show the risk of regaining weight after withdrawing from the medication are quite high. The majority of people who stop taking semaglutide regain two-thirds of the weight they lost while on the drug within just one year! This means you may need to be on the medication for life to sustain results.

If, after speaking with a medical professional, you decide to take the injections, the dietary recommendations in this book still apply.

Whether you take the drug for life or opt for intermittent usage, the weight loss injection should be used as a tool to make healthy eating easier and support sustainable health outcomes. I highly recommend working with a registered dietitian to ensure you're eating properly on a weight loss drug.

Should I Fast?

Fasting is defined as not eating for a period of time. It can regulate blood sugar levels, improve the gut microbiome, and decrease risk of

---

[8] *I interviewed Obesity Medicine Specialist Dr. Nikita Shah on episode #163 of The Nutrition Awareness Podcast. Check it out for more information about what drugs like Ozempic are (and what they are not), what to expect, and how to safely utilize them.*

chronic disease . Because we all fast when we sleep, I encourage most of my clients to fast for 12-13 hours each night at least five days per week. This is known as Circadian Fasting, which implies not eating while the sun is down.

An example of a 13-hour Circadian fast would be eating dinner at 6 p.m. and not eating another bite until breakfast at 7 AM. If you eat dinner at 7:30 p.m. the following day, you can push breakfast to 8:30 AM. Water will not break your fast and should be consumed upon waking. Wait to do any intense exercise until after you've broken your fast.

Women interested in fasting should refer to the book "Fast Like a Girl" by Dr. Mindy Pelz. She's a pioneer in researching fasting according to a woman's cycle.

Ready, Set, Go!

Now that we've reviewed the BNT Protocol and answered common nutrition questions, it's time I introduce you to the first of six of my All-or-Nothing clients and their stories. Please refer back to Part 1 of this book as often as you need to make sense of the nutrition recommendations throughout each chapter. Let's do this!

Part 2

Chapter 1
The Food Tracker

Shadow Tendencies:

- Counts calories

- Tracks macronutrients

- Weighs food

- Only feels "safe" around food when it's being tracked

- Obsesses over body measurements such as weight or waist circumferences

- Restarts the same diet (face it, they're all diets) over and over but expects different results

- Stresses when there are no calorie counts on a menu

- Classifies food as "good" or "bad"

- Restricts food or calories during the week, but "cheats" on weekends or at special events

- Struggles with consistency

Food Tracking Works... Until it Doesn't

"I hope you won't judge me for drinking such a colossal coffee," my newest client Claire, age 33, admitted as she settled in for our first of many 8 AM appointments. "I was so anxious for today, I barely slept. I need the caffeine."

To assure her my office was a judgment-free zone, I tipped the lid of my trash can and revealed my empty Starbucks cup. We shared a laugh over our espresso dependency, but I could tell Claire was uncomfortable. She fiddled with the ends of her sleek black side braid and shifted around in her seat like a suspect being interrogated. If she wore any make-up, it was as subtle as the thin line of sweat on her forehead. A comfortable 75-degree Fahrenheit December day in Florida, it couldn't have been the humidity.

Despite the sunshine outside, Claire's frame was swallowed by a beige sweatshirt and loose black joggers. I wondered if by dressing in baggy clothes, she was trying to hide her weight. From what I could see, Claire was of average height—about 5'5"—and nowhere near obese though she had soft & feminine features. Her almond-shaped eyes, porcelain skin, and curve of her cheeks reflected her Chinese American heritage. Her ankles were crossed, her feet sporting a pair of bright white Air Force Ones. I resisted the impulse to ask her how she managed to keep her sneakers so squeaky clean as I couldn't take a step out the door without smudging my soles with dirt and grime.

"I wasn't sure what information you needed from me, so I brought everything I had," Claire announced, interrupting my thoughts.

She whipped out an oversized binder from her Louis Vuitton Neverfull bag, set it on my desk, and cracked open the cover. Inside were seven color-coded tabs organizing her papers and photos. Within each section were pages of food diaries dating from 2012, workout plans, charts documenting her weight history, and lengthy lists of vitamins and supplements.

Impressive? Yes. Excessive? Very.

"There's also three years' worth of blood test results from my primary care physician," Claire continued as she thumbed through the pages. "For the past six years, my hormone panels and labs have been normal. I included them in the back if you'd like to review them."

I didn't have the heart to tell Claire I didn't need to see her pre-pandemic cholesterol levels, nor was I going to take time to read through her old food logs. Since our time together was limited to an hour, I wanted to get into the juicy stuff as soon as possible.

Prior to our appointment, I asked Claire to fill out an intake form that included her goals for our session. Like most of my first-time clients, she had answered: *I want to lose weight and feel better.*

Her vague response gave me very little to work with. What does *feel better* mean? Is it improved energy, confidence, or mood? Did she want her favorite pair of jeans to fit less snug or did she want to completely transform her physique? I needed more detail, so I asked Claire to expand on why she was in my office.

"Ever since I turned 30, my old approach to weight loss doesn't work," she started, sounding as deflated as a soufflé. "It used to be easy for me. After a vacation or cheat day, I'd simply count calories and drop the pounds without issues."

I winced at the term c*heat day.* Calling a meal a "cheat" reminded me of Catholic guilt but for diets. A weekend of conveniently forgetting the religious demands of diet culture followed by a week of shame and Hail Marys in the form of chalky protein bars or skipped meals? No thanks.

Claire continued. "I tried counting macronutrients, but that isn't working either. Not only do I feel confused about which foods are good or bad for me, I don't know if I am eating too much or too little. My friends have pointed out my preoccupation with food has become obsessive and encouraged me to seek help. I need someone to guide me on how to approach this whole weight loss thing so I can feel like myself again."

"Which means...?"

"Feeling confident," Claire answered without skipping a beat, "about how I look *and* how I eat. I want to look in the mirror without nitpicking all of my imperfections, then trying to correct them by obsessively tracking what I eat. I used to be able to walk out of the house in a sleeveless dress, but now I refuse to wear my old summer clothes because I'm too insecure about my arms. It'd also be nice to snack without mentally tallying up every single bite so I can record it later. Enjoying a healthy meal without questioning what the calorie count is would be nice."

For Claire to feel good in her skin, she needed to break free from her preoccupation with controlling her food intake. She needed to learn how to look at the big picture so she could plan healthy meals and make the right choices on the fly. In the following months, she'd practice eating without tracking until she felt assured in her decision-making. I anticipated her self-image would improve alongside her confidence around food.

Your Turn

Pretend you're making an appointment with a Registered Dietitian and are asked to describe your ultimate health goals. If you could get everything you wanted a year from now, what would be different about how you feel, eat, or look? What's your ideal wellness routine look like? Are there improvements in your energy levels or confidence? How about your medications or blood labs (cholesterol, blood sugars, etc)? Include any fitness goals as well.

Revisit this vision throughout the book to help you set meaningful goals and stay on a healthy path!

Based on her history, it was clear Claire was a seasoned dieter. Her years of counting calories, obsessing over her food, and repeating the same macro-tracking diet multiple times fit the sub-archetype **The Food Tracker**.

Your Turn

Answer the following questions. Do you...

1. Obsess over the   calories in a food or meal?

2. Frequently use calorie or macronutrient counting applications?

3. Attempt calorie-restricted diets?

4. Count macronutrient intake each day (commonly referred as *counting macros*)?

5. Give up on calorie or macronutrient counting as soon as you mess up and overeat?

6. Feel upset with yourself when you don't "hit your macros" or calorie goals?

7. Restart the same calorie or macro-counting diets over and over?

8. Choose low calorie menu options, even if you want something else?

9. Prioritize the calories or macronutrients in a diet over how the food tastes, satisfies, or makes you feel?

10. See foods as "good" or "bad"?

11. Feel guilty when you don't eat "clean"?

12. Track your weight, body measurements, or body fat percentage obsessively?

13. Base your self-worth or progress on the results of the above?

14. Plan cheat meals that turn into a string of cheat days?

If you answered "yes" to three or more of these questions, you may identify with shadow tendencies of The Food Tracker sub-archetype. The strategies in this chapter will help you learn to trust yourself to eat without counting calories, macros, or weighing food.

Does Mother Know Best?

"It sounds like you've followed a lot of programs that encourage you to measure your food and track everything you eat," I said after Claire answered yes to nearly all of the of the questions above.

"Is that... wrong?"

"Is it?"

Claire's dark brown eyes twitched. I changed the subject.

"You mentioned you're confused and obsessive about food. Let's start there. How old were you when those feelings first arose?"

"If I am being honest, food has been a stress point for as long as I can remember," Claire sighed. "My mom was the kind of woman who would just eat a handful of raw almonds when she felt hungry, whereas I have a big appetite. After school, she'd shake her head when I had snacks before dinner and mumble *Tān chī guǐ*, which translates to *greedy eater*. I ate because I was genuinely hungry after running around at recess and P.E. class, not because I was greedy."

I imagined Claire as a little 4th grader on the school bus going home, looking forward to an afternoon snack but knowing her mom would disapprove. It must have been confusing to be shamed for being hungry.

"As I've gotten older, the comments have gotten harsher," Claire continued. "Last week, she screenshotted a photo of me I posted on Instagram saying I was too chubby to be wearing a dress so tight."

She pulled out her phone to show me. In the post, Claire was flaunting fitted black midi length dress highlighting her subtle yet feminine curves, soft arms, and strong calves. I thought she looked fabulous, but a critical eye will body shame anyone, including supermodels.

"Right?" Claire's slouched back in her chair, melting into the fabric like a snowman on a sunny day. "My mom is the daughter of a first-generation immigrant from China. In her culture, it's acceptable to comment on women's bodies and appetites."

"What about your dad?" I asked.

"He thankfully doesn't say much about my weight," Claire said. "He's Caucasian, if that matters. My mom and dad divorced when I was 6, and they have both remarried."

Regardless of cultural background, it's not uncommon for me to hear stories from individuals about parents making judgmental remarks regarding their eating habits, food choices, bodies, or serving sizes. Older generations were raised to believe being a size two with a flat tummy was the pinnacle of beauty and normalized outlandish diets such as *The Cabbage Soup Diet[9]*. Many women have not realized (or are unwilling to recognize) unrealistic beauty standards and fad diets can be harmful, especially to women with naturally curvier builds.

I suspect parents who make passive aggressive comments about their daughters' eating habits are projecting their own food and body insecurities. If a maternal guardian values thinness, she may micro-manage her daughter's diet because she feels out of control with food herself. This kind of mom (commonly referred to as an *Almond Mom[10]*) may attribute the trauma of her teenage years to her weight, thinking life would have been easier if she were a size 2 and not a 10. In a twisted effort to protect her daughter from the same pain she felt, mom attempts to control what her kid eats by serving only the most natural, healthy foods.

If mom was a size 2 and was praised for having a smaller body, she may believe it's the only acceptable way to exist. She'll disguise her criticism of her daughter's body as concern so she can justify restrictive eating practices.

---

[9] *The cabbage soup diet, popular in the 50's and 60's, involves consuming large amounts of cabbage soup for seven days. Proponents thought since the soup is low in calories and high in fiber, it could lead to feelings of fullness and therefore, weight loss. It is not recommended for long-term results.*

[10] *Coined from social media in 2023, the derogatory term 'Almond Mom' refers to a mother who is overly concerned with her child's health. She often takes extreme measures to make sure her kids are served the most natural ingredients and is strict about eating only healthy food.*

In both scenarios, moms are mistakenly basing a woman's worth on her weight and approaching health from a disordered lens. Any way you frame it, shaming a child or teenager's eating habits can permanently scar her relationship with food and body.

Mothers are their children's first and primary example of what it means to be a woman. If young girls see mom pinching the jiggle of her arms or opting for a glass of water when she's hungry, young girls will do the same because they think that's just what women do! Unless moms actively monitor how they speak of food or their figure in front of their families, girls will inherit the fear of eating and mimic the same hateful remarks about their bodies.

"I can't help feeling some resentment towards my mom," Claire confessed. "I'm certain I would not have so many struggles with my weight and body image if she hadn't been so critical."

"I don't blame you for feeling that way," I affirmed. "Your mom most likely was doing the best she could, but that doesn't mean her words were not harmful. Have you ever talked to her about how her attitude around body image and food impacted you?"

Claire looked away and cracked her knuckles, eliciting a series of popping noises that sounded like bubble gum. "No. Even if I did, it wouldn't matter. She's not receptive to talking about feelings or concerns about body image. Which reminds me, my family is hosting a Lunar New Year's party in a couple of months. I know my mom is going to comment on my weight before she even says *hello*."

I flinched. "Yikes."

"What really stinks is how there will be *so* much delicious food. Beef dumplings, crispy spring rolls, and noodle soup…" Claire's gaze fell to the floor. "I wish I were looking forward to the meal, but the whole ordeal stresses me out. Not only am I worried about all the calories in the food, but my family takes offense when I don't eat second or third helpings. One minute they're telling me I'm too fat, the next they're questioning why I left food on my plate. I just can't win."

Your Turn

1. Reflect on your primary caregiver's relationship with food and body image. Did they diet, make comments about their own body or eating habits, or gossip about the weights or diets of others?

2. Consider if this person impacted your relationship with food and body image. Was their influence negative, positive, or neutral?

3. Pretend you could change anything about how this person spoke about or behaved around food. What would you change? How would those changes shape your own relationship with food and your body?

4. If you're a parent, do your answers reflect how you're speaking about food to your children? If not, what needs to change so you don't pass down the same food and body image struggles to your kids?

Good & Bad Foods

"What if your mom was wrong? Maybe you didn't have a big appetite, just a normal one," I suggested to Claire.

"I've never considered that," Claire said, her red-polished finger lightly pressing her cheek. "I'm not sure what normal is, but I doubt my mom knows, either."

"As a kid, how did your mother's comments about your plate affect you?"

"I'm a certified people-pleaser, so I tried to fit the mold of what she considered acceptable, but honestly, I only ate *'good'* when she watched me. When I was on my own or with my friends, I'd eat whatever I wanted in massive portions. Milkshakes, Danishes, fettuccine Alfredo... all the bad carbs!"

Claire's secretive eating was not surprising. When people suppress their appetites at meal times in an effort to follow a diet or expectation, it often leads to eating in secret (more on this in **The Perfectionist**).

In Claire's mind, high calorie foods like creamy pasta were "bad" while low calorie foods like carrots were "good." She was a black and white thinker when it came to eating, which left no room for flexibility. This mentality is not uncommon with all-or-nothing dieters like Claire, and it's a habit we'd have to nip in the bud if she wanted to stop feeling miserable around food.

Unfortunately, all of the misinformation on the internet can cause paranoia around every food on the planet. Take a banana, for instance. One article frames a banana as a healthy pre-portioned snack packed with B vitamins and fiber while another claims it's a sugar stick with too many carbohydrates. Damned if you and damned if you don't!

Obsessed with the morality and calorie content of food, Food Trackers like Claire do not stop to question how foods make them *feel* after eating. A banana can taste good and give them energy to run a 5k race, but they make their decisions based on their daily caloric or carbohydrate budget.

I once had a client named Helen who would track her calories perfectly until dinner when she ate whatever her wife whipped up. Not wanting to record any foods that were not "clean," Helen would stop counting for the day and serve herself as much as she wanted. Knowing she already ate over her daily allowance, she'd say, *Screw it, already messed up,* and munch on kettle popcorn and cocoa-dusted nuts through the evening.

"At least popcorn and nuts aren't as bad as chips, right?" Helen tried to justify.

By attaching morality to foods, Helen gave herself an excuse to overeat them. Once the snacks were out, she'd feel guilty about not tracking and vow to do better the next day. Not surprisingly, the next day was rarely any different.

When I shared Helen's story with Claire, she told me it was familiar. "It's not uncommon for me to overeat after my allotted food ran out during the day. Like Helen, I use it as a reason to keep eating."

"Do you tell yourself you'll do better tomorrow?"

"Always," Claire chuckled. "I tell myself it's the last time, so I might as well enjoy whatever I want!"

Claire's resistance to incorporating "bad" foods such as jelly pastries or queso-smothered burritos into her usual diet fueled a scarcity mindset. By forbidding certain foods, they became harder to resist. As soon as she gave in to temptation, Claire's brain justified this as "bad" behavior. She would tell herself, *This will be the last time* or *I won't eat sugar again for a month!* These kinds of thoughts gave her permission to eat as much as she wanted, commonly known as *The Last Supper Mentality*[11]. As counterintuitive it may seem, detaching morality from food would help Claire feel less guilty about what she ate.

I asked Claire to share with me a list of her favorite forbidden foods.

"Oh, where do I begin?! I love Sour Patch Kids, cheese fries, chocolate bars, breakfast pastries…" Claire spouted, her face lit like a front porch light on a gloomy night. "And popcorn chicken. I love to top a bowl of buttery mashed potatoes and gravy with fried chicken!"

"While I don't want you to eat buckets of fried chicken and bags of sour candy for breakfast, I don't want you to classify these foods as bad or restrict them entirely," I chuckled. "Instead, combine healthy foods per the BNT Protocol with these foods. If you'd normally eat a bowl of creamy pasta, add grilled shrimp or broccoli. You'll feel fuller on less pasta because you're adding protein and fiber from nutritious foods."

Claire's eyes widened. "You mean, I'm allowed to eat pasta?"

"Sure," I said. "Since that will help you get rid of *The Last Supper Mentality,* eat it as part of a balanced, nutritious diet."

"How do I do that?"

Since Claire was a **Food Tracker**, she needed to leverage her need for structure by pre-planning how she could include these once forbidden foods into her diet without tracking every bite.

"The first step is following the BNT Protocol," I said. "This means planning and choosing balanced and nutritious foods that you enjoy throughout the day. When at least 80% or more of your diet follows the BNT Protocol, you can feel confident that you're on a healthy path.

---

[11] *The "Last Supper Mentality" is a term to describe overindulging before beginning a restrictive eating pattern. The name comes from the Christian tradition of The Last Supper, a final meal shared by Jesus Christ and his disciples before he was crucified.*

If you have an appetite for forbidden foods, you'll be able to eat them without having a Last Supper Mentality."

"Can you give me examples?" Claire asked.

I pulled out a list of common forbidden foods with examples on how to integrate them into a balanced, healthy diet

Forbidden Food	Healthy Integration
Peanut butter	Add a scoop to old-fashioned oatmeal with berries and cinnamon Make a nutritious PB&J with a seedy bread and whole berries instead of jelly
Creamy Pasta	Stir in roasted veggies and turkey meatballs for more protein and fiber Use a high-fiber version such as chickpea pasta or whole wheat
Bagels	Toast a whole wheat bagel and top with avocado and eggs instead of cream cheese or sugary spread
Soda	Sip at the movies or during long road trips, along with a balanced meal or snack
Fresh Baked Cookies and Brownies	Eat alongside Greek yogurt and fruit Enjoy after a protein-rich meal

Table 2.1.1

Using the list, Claire brainstormed ideas on how she could integrate forbidden foods. By anticipating a savory slice of coffee cake with her eggs on Sunday, a small piece of hazelnut chocolate after a healthy work lunch, and a side order of cheese fries to split with her bowling league teammates, she would feel less restricted and more in control. Later in our session, we would integrate these plans into a weekly meal calendar.

Your Turn

List forbidden foods you restrict but find yourself periodically overeating. Using the BNT Protocol and Table 2.1.1, choose at least three of these foods and plan how to include them within your balanced diet.

Forbidden Food	Healthy Integration

Old Habits Die-*t* Hard

"I'm equal parts excited and nervous about integrating forbidden foods into my diet," Claire confessed. "I've had The Last Supper Mentality for as long as I can remember, and eating without tracking calories feels scary."

"When did you first start counting calories?" I asked.

"I lightly dieted in high school, but it got out of control in college."

"How so?"

"I'd eat healthy for a few days, but when I went out with friends, I'd stuff my face with wings, fries, and beer. College was my first taste of freedom—figuratively and literally. When I came home after first semester, I had put on tons of weight and of course, my mom noticed." Claire laughed half-heartedly but her expression remained serious. I wondered if she used humor to lessen the pain she felt about her mom's judgment. "Shortly after, I stumbled upon an Instagram fitness model sharing before and after pictures of her clients on her social media platform. She was boasting about their dramatic fat loss in just 8-weeks using her *Fat to Fit* meal plan and workout program."

Fat to Fit? I thought. The cringey name screamed 2010's diet culture. Like many people who are eager to lose weight, reading exaggerated testimonials from participants of *Fat to Fit* prompted Claire to sign up without thinking twice. She was desperate to lose weight, so she didn't consider the long-term repercussions of dieting.

I asked Claire to tell me about the *Fat to Fit* program.

"I can show you!" Claire flipped to a tab in her binder labeled *F2F*. I couldn't believe Claire still had printouts of her meal plan along with food diaries tallying her daily calorie and macro counts. During the program, Claire also documented every workout, which included five strength training sessions and two **high intensity interval training (HIIT)**[12] workouts each week.

I looked at what the plan instructed Claire to eat every Monday for 8 weeks:

---

[12] *HIIT workouts involve several rounds of quick movements that increase the heart rate to at least 80% of one's max heart rate followed by equally short periods of rest or low intensity movements.*

Fat to Fit Meal Plan: Monday

Time	Food
6 a.m. breakfast	1 cup egg whites, 1 slice toast Black coffee, unlimited
9 a.m. post-workout	1 scoop whey protein powder with water or 8 ounces of unsweetened almond milk
12 p.m. lunch	4 ounces grilled chicken 1 cup raw spinach with 1/2 tbsp of extra virgin olive oil 1/2 cup cooked broccoli 1/2 cup cooked brown rice
3 p.m. snack	¼ cup almonds or a protein bar
6 p.m. dinner	4 ounces tilapia 1 cup cooked asparagus 4 ounces cooked sweet potato
8 p.m. snack	1 scoop whey protein powder with water or 8 ounces unsweetened almond milk

Yikes, I thought. This had to be one of the most unappetizing diets I'd witnessed (and I had seen a lot).

Claire's macronutrient records revealed she was eating large amounts of protein, low amounts of carbohydrate, and not enough dietary fat. Even worse, her total caloric intake was between 1200-1300 calories per day. This was *much* lower than what I'd recommend for an active adult woman. In fact, most toddlers and large dogs require 1200-1400 calories per day. Claire was not a toddler and certainly not a dog.

Not surprisingly, most of Claire's meals were stereotypical of "clean eating" programs: lots of broccoli, chicken, and brown rice or tilapia with sweet potato and steamed asparagus. She guzzled two whey protein shakes each day and sometimes chugged egg whites for breakfast. Gross!

In my experience, proponents of "clean eating" take nutrition to extremes. They demonize foods that are not *pure*, *whole*, or *natural*. These terms are not regulated by the Food and Drug Administration (FDA), so what is allowed on a clean eating diet can get misconstrued. For instance, organic hummus may be considered "clean" by one person but "processed" by another. The language confuses people like Claire, and because the lines are so blurred, many clean eaters have an undiagnosed form of orthorexia, an eating disorder that involves an unhealthy obsession with healthy eating. Women with orthorexia constantly worry about whether their food is acceptable or not, leading to feelings of anxiety, social isolation, and body dysmorphia. In extreme cases, individuals with orthorexia can suffer from hair loss, dry skin, low blood pressure, digestive concerns such as constipation and bloating, dehydration, anemia, and malnutrition. I suspected Claire's mother had a form of orthorexia.

During the *Fat to Fit* program, Claire would plan one meal per week where she threw all her clean eating rules out the window and ate whatever she wanted in one sitting with no tracking. She called trips to the sushi buffet cheat meals, but I considered them binge eating episodes. A binge eating episode is when an individual consumes large quantities of food in a short time span. While **The Binge Eater** chapter provides more detail, binge eating is different from overeating because there is an inability to control one's portions or stop eating at the point of physical discomfort. Ironically, binge eating commonly becomes a problem while someone is dieting.

Claire proceeded to show me photos of her body transformation using the *Fit to Fat* method. Her weight loss was pretty dramatic. She had lost 23 pounds in two months. While the media would portray Claire's transformation as a success story, I viewed it as self-induced starvation and a recipe for disaster.

"After the eight weeks were up, I decided to keep tracking in my food tracker app. If anything, I became more extreme," Claire admitted.

"I began to weigh food and refused to eat anything without the calories or macronutrient listed. After a month, I lost five more pounds!"

Claire was able to maintain this weight until she went on vacation to Italy with her sorority. As soon as she got home, she felt defeated by how much she had eaten during her trip and stopped tracking. Within a year, she had gained all of the weight back and then some.

"I've tried to restart the plan at least six or seven times but each time I try, I fail within weeks," Claire whined. "I can't seem to get the same results as the first time around, and I'm over it."

Heck yes, I thought. *She's open to a new approach!*

"I need accountability to stay on track. I want someone to tell me exactly what and how much to eat so I stop falling off the wagon."

Okay, never mind.

I quickly realized Claire's experience losing weight using a strict meal plan had led her to believe tracking every gram of food she put in her mouth was the only way to be successful. She also was under the impression that someone else should dictate how she ate instead of listening to own body. Because Claire's mom shamed her for being hungry and monitored her eating habits, Claire never learned to trust herself with food. We were going to change that!

I decided to ask open-ended questions to help her recognize how obsessive food tracking was driving a wedge between her and a healthy relationship to food.

"I heard you say you have tried tracking what you eat multiple times. What happens to make you stop?"

"The weekend," Claire chuckled. "Or some unexpected plans that involve bad foods. As soon as a wrench is thrown in my week, I give up entirely."

"Then what?" I asked, suspecting her answer to be…

"I start my diet over on Monday."

Monday Blues

Ah, Monday. Restarting a diet after the weekend, the 1st of the month, or following a vacation is a classic Food Tracker move. Food Trackers tell themselves it's ok to order the loaded Philly cheesesteak because they'll eat salad tomorrow. It's a convenient scapegoat for breaking their own rules. They're not technically giving up—they're just pro-crastinating... *eye roll!*

In reality, "starting over on Monday" is an excuse to eat whatever all weekend without guilt. So is saying, "I've eaten healthy all week, so I deserve this cheat." By dividing the week into *good* and *bad* days, Food Trackers continue to circle aimlessly through the clouded smoke of a destructive diet culture vortex.

To be successful for the long haul, Food Trackers must let go of the idea that their week is ruined because of one spontaneous dessert or meal out. Instead of saying, *I'll start over on Monday,* they must think, *The next meal is a new opportunity to pick up where I left off.*

When Food Trackers begin planning a balanced diet that includes room for flexibility, they will no longer need start and stop dates. Even if they eat barbecued ribs and coleslaw for lunch on Saturday, they will eat something more balanced for dinner such as a tofu stir fry or chickpea pasta salad for dinner.

Your Turn

Do you use Mondays (or specific start dates) as an excuse to eat whatever you want? Is it helpful, or is it an excuse to eat whatever you want during the weekend?

Creating Structure

"I feel so called out!" Claire joked. "I definitely use Monday as an excuse to eat whatever I want. In college, it was easier for me to limit my cheats to a single meal but these days, one meal turns into an entire weekend. I'm not sure why."

"What was different about your life then versus now?" I asked.

"A lot," Claire laughed. "Back then, I didn't have much of a life out-side of studying, work, and the gym. All I cared about was having the perfect body, perfect grades, and perfect resume. My social life took a backseat. Now I'm in a long-term relationship and have a solid group of friends. We like to bowl, explore theme parks, and take weekend trips to the beach. All of that socializing makes it hard to stick to any diet."

"Sounds like your life is a lot more exciting these days."

"Maybe too exciting. We eat out almost every meal during the weekend, and it's never anything healthy. You know the character Violet from *Charlie and the Chocolate Factory*? The one who turns into a giant blueberry? That's how I feel on Sundays. I need to be more disciplined on the weekends."

Claire didn't require more discipline. What Claire needed was a fresh perspective and a new approach to eating. Instead of trying to fight against her body like it was the enemy, Claire needed to realize she and her body were one and the same. Diets were disturbing the peace Claire needed to foster with her body so she could prosper!

"It's time to send your *Fat To Fit Meal Plan* through the paper shredder," I declared. "Using the BNT Protocol, you're going to begin eating more balanced meals in the week and planning for flexibility when you want it."

"The BNT Protocol makes perfect sense to me," she started, peering at The BNT Protocol handouts I gave her. "But if I am not following a plan, it's hard for me to trust myself around food. I'm afraid if I let myself eat more on the weekdays, I'll still overdo it and end up gaining weight."

I understood her perspective. Like a toddler letting go of his old and torn baby blanket even though it's no longer functional, it still provides comfort. Claire was no different. After spending years of her life following diets, it was overwhelming to leave the false sense of security behind.

A good dietitian understands that it's in a Food Tracker's nature to need plans and structure to thrive. When Food Trackers are lost in their shadow side, these obsessive tendencies can get out of control and cause more damage than good. But with awareness, Food Trackers can leverage their need for data and order in productive ways. As a result, they'll learn how to eat based on their own needs and lessen their dependence on fad diets and calorie counter applications.

To do so, I prescribe two tools for Food Trackers like Claire: *Meal Planning* and *Food, Mood, and Body Journals*.

Meal Planning

Claire only felt confident about her choices when she obeyed the laws of a cookie cutter meal plan that spoon-fed her what, how much, and when to eat. As soon as she broke a rule, she threw caution to the wind, eating whatever was convenient and sounded tasty. As a result, she made no lasting progress.

"Without a preset meal plan, I feel overwhelmed by grocery shopping," Claire confessed. "I buy a bunch of vegetables but don't know what to do with them, so I order take-out or make choices I regret because I'm in a pinch."

It was time for Claire to set goals around planning meals. While this required more work up front, creating her own menu following the BNT Protocol would help her stay accountable for the long haul. Planning and prepping would also make her inner Food Tracker feel safe, allowing her to stay consistent with a less restrictive approach. Plus, she'd get to eat more foods she enjoyed!

In a similar scenario, my neighbor and eventual client Ellie lost weight following a meal plan she got from her personal trainer but couldn't maintain the progress because she hated the food he instructed her to eat.

"I'm tired of everything on this damn list," Ellie complained, scrunching her nose in disgust. "Plus, I feel like an oddball at meals. Everyone's eating spaghetti and meatballs while I'm stuck with the same ol' baked cod. My oldest son pokes fun at my plate, calling it *Mommy's stinky fish*."

Using the BNT Protocol, we adjusted Ellie's meal plan to add more variety and flavor. Instead of a heaping bowl of noodles, she planned to eat lean chicken meatballs she prepared for both her and the entire family and kept the spaghetti as a side dish. Rather than devouring half a loaf of garlic bread, she savored one piece with an arugula green salad dressed in olive oil, chickpeas, and lemon juice.

By planning ahead, Ellie was able to envision a variety of balanced meals she actually enjoyed, control her portions, include more veggies, and not have to cook two separate meals for her family.

Other benefits to meal planning that Ellie noticed included:

1. Choosing recipes that matched her culinary skill level

2. Swapping ingredients for ones that matched her dietary preferences and restrictions

3. Planning ahead for special occasions and meals out

4. Doubling or tripling recipes for the following day's lunch or dinner

"The best part is not having to stress about what to eat each week," Ellie told me. "Once the planning is done, it's smooth sailing."

I shared these benefits to Claire, then advised her to give it a try. "For beginners, meal planning is best completed on a weekly basis. I recommend using a 7-day calendar with at least four rows: breakfast, lunch, dinner, and snacks. For each day of the week, write in what you plan to eat."

"Could I use a meal planner on my phone?" asked Claire.

"While there are many digital meal calendar apps, I encourage new meal planners to rely on pen and paper," I replied. "Writing it on a tangible sheet allows you to hang it in your kitchen so your meal plan is front and center."

"Good point," Claire said. "It's not uncommon for me to download an app just to forget about it."

"You're not alone!" I assured her. "While you can search for any meal planning template online, let me show you the calendar I use. Then, I'll share the five steps I take to complete it."

nutrition
awareness

MEAL PLANNER

	SUN	MON	TUE	WED	THU	FRI	SAT
MEAL 1							
MEAL 2							
MEAL 3							
MEAL 4							
WORK-OUT							

Download and print the same calendar I use with my clients by going to: www.kaitrichardsonrd.com

5 Steps to Meal Planning

Step 1: Plan for Meals Out

Anticipating meals saves on food waste and grocery bills. If lunch on Tuesday is with friends and Fridays are reserved for date night, there's no need to buy or prepare food for those days.

Having a visual of how many meals you plan to eat out each week can encourage more home cooking and healthy decision making. Simply seeing that there are already three meals reserved for special occasions can motivate you to skip ordering take-out during more mundane meals.

Step 2: Collect Recipes

With so many healthy recipes online, the possibilities of what to cook are endless! I recommend clients with less experience in the kitchen start by specifying *easy* or *simple* in their search. If time is an issue, look up recipes that are *quick* or *20 minutes or less*.

When selecting a recipe, consider the following:

- Is the recipe balanced with protein, carbohydrates, and healthy fats?

- Are there fruits and vegetables, or will you need to add them?

- Are 80% of the ingredients nutritious per the BNT Protocol?

- Which cooking utensils and appliances are necessary?

- How much total prep and cook time will it take?

- How many servings does each recipe make?

- Does the recipe actually look good?

I've included my favorite recipes on my website: www.kaitrichardsonrd.com.

Pro tip: *Check ingredients you may have in your pantry and fridge, then seek out recipes that utilize these ingredients. Have a bag of frozen* *edamame in the freezer? Google* Healthy Lunch with Edamame *to see what you can find.*

Step 3: Schedule Meals

Plan which days to prep and eat each recipe.

Step 4: Make a List

Write a grocery list of the ingredients required for each meal or snack. If you're prepping one recipe for multiple meals, double check how many servings each recipe produces—you may need to double up on some ingredients!

Once you have your list, go back and scratch off ingredients you already have in your kitchen so you don't overbuy or waste food. If there are foods you don't like in your recipes, look up alternatives.

Don't be afraid to buy ready-to-eat versions of ingredients such as grains, proteins, or veggies. There is no shame in buying steamed produce or pre-seasoned meat if it gets you to make a healthier choice.

Step 5: Shop!

Make time to hit the store or use a grocery delivery app to get what you need. You can do one major grocery haul each week or make multiple smaller trips to the store. I like to do one trip to a major grocery chain where I get 80-90% of what I need, then another one midweek to stock up on little things from specialty food shops.

Your Turn

Following the five steps, plan your meals for the next week. If planning three meals for every day of the week feels overwhelming, start by planning just breakfast or lunch for 3-4 days a week.

Making Meal Planning a Habit

Meal planning one time isn't helpful if it does not become routine. Since Claire had a busy work and social life, she needed to commit to a day and time to write out her meals. Even if she wasn't ready to pre-prep the food, organizing was non-negotiable if she wanted to be successful.

"I know the popular day to prepare meals is Sunday, but I hate wasting a weekend on grocery shopping," Claire confessed. "Can I do it another time?"

"There is no right or wrong way to organize your weekly eats, as long as planning and prepping becomes a habit," I responded.

Shamella, one of my very first clients, planned and ordered her week's groceries while she waited in the pick-up line at her kids' school on Fridays. At first, it felt tedious and time-consuming, but after a few weeks of consistent meal planning, Shamella had become incredibly efficient. Soon, she was planning her family of five's entire menu within 30 minutes.

My friend Hannah went to pilates every Saturday. After her class, she'd walk next door to a coffee shop and plan her work lunches for the next week. Once she finished, she'd swing by the grocery store on the way home and pick up her ingredients. It worked like a charm!

I asked Claire if any of these examples sparked inspiration. She told me shopping after work on Monday worked well for her but planning for the whole week in one sitting felt daunting.

"By Thursday, I don't want to eat what I've bought or prepped," she groaned. "Either the produce has gone bad, or I'm not in the mood to eat what I planned. I mean, how am I supposed to know on Monday what I'll crave on Friday?"

"You make a good point, but you know your own preferences better than everyone else, right?"

"Right."

"Then you have three options," I said matter-of-factly. "Option one, plan something you predict you'll enjoy and stick to it no matter what."

"You're saying if I planned baked cod and asparagus but crave nachos, eat the cod anyway?"

"Exactly."

Claire let out a huff.

"I know it can be challenging, but no one regrets eating up their healthy groceries after the fact. Stick to your plan and plan to eat nachos another night."

Claire shot me a look that said, *I hear you but I'm not happy about it.* "What is option two?"

"Instead of planning seven days at once, divide your meal planning into two separate sessions. Plan and shop on Monday, then again on Thursday."

"All of this feels like a lot of work," she grumbled. "Is the third option easier?"

"The third option is to ignore all my recommendations, continue eating as you have been, and stall your health progress. Seems like a waste of time and money, don't ya think?"

Many people want to change, but they don't want to grow because growing takes time, energy, and sacrifice. It's easier to print a meal plan offline, follow it for a week, then revert to ordering UberEats every night. If Claire wanted to turn a new leaf, she needed to make time to learn how to eat, plan healthy meals, and get in the kitchen. I knew that in time, it would become habitual.

"Alright, alright," Claire sighed. "I hear ya'. Every Thursday evening from 6-8 p.m., I play in a bowling league. I can make a mini meal plan after work and stop by Trader Joe's on the way home."

I let out a little cheer. Claire had the self-awareness to realize she was more likely to follow through with meal planning if she broke it into chunks while Shamella and Hannah found success with one weekly haul. Whatever works, *works.*

As I stood up to grab copies of the meal planner, I asked Claire if she ever ate dinner at the bowling alley. Although I hadn't been to a bowling alley since an awkward first date years ago, I could only assume the menu didn't offer options besides nachos with goopy, liquid cheese and buckets of light beer.

"Um, yes." Claire's fair cheeks grew as pink as the aperture of an aged conch shell. "It's embarrassing, but our team name is the *Cereal Bowls,* so we take turns bringing in boxes of cereal and jugs of milk to share. I know it's bad, but it's fun to try the craziest flavors. Last week,

I brought blueberry pancake flavored cereal puffs! I guess I have to give those up, huh?"

"Not necessarily," I suggested as I stuck a giant paper clip over a stack of meal planner print-outs, leaving out one sheet for us to practice on. "Would your team disown you if you brought a healthier dinner to eat alongside a smaller cup of the sugary cereal?"

Instead of banishing cereal to the lost land of forbidden foods, I wanted her to have full permission to enjoy whatever she wanted. That way, Claire wouldn't feel restricted and subsequently tempted to overeat when she "cheated." But foods like sugary cereal aren't always filling on their own, so eating a nutritious meal alongside, or before, a treat would help her feel in control of her choices and portions.

"They'd tease me, but it's nothing I can't take," Claire smirked. "Any suggestions on what to bring?"

Racking my brain for something healthy yet socially acceptable to eat in a bowling alley, I pictured Claire munching on a kale citrus salad surrounded by men dressed in polos slurping fountain sodas and wiping the pizza grease from their fingers. For her to fit in, anything with vegetables had to be disguised.

"How about a whole grain buffalo chicken wrap stuffed with slaw and Greek yogurt dressing? Or an egg salad made with avocados instead of mayo?"

Snatching the pen from my hands, she scribbled *Buff Wrap* in the meal planner's Thursday dinner slot.

Your Turn

Each week, which days and times can you carve out at least 90 minutes to meal plan, shop, and/or order groceries? If planning for 7 days in one sitting is too much, can you split this planning and shopping process into two or three different sessions?

Empathetic Eating

I once had a client Lisa tell me she was an Empathetic Eater at work. When I asked her to explain, Lisa said she often found herself eating baked goods she didn't like or want because someone at the office made them for her and she didn't want to hurt their feelings. Her best friend in the office complained about their boss over appetizers and spinach artichoke dip, and Lisa felt bad ordering something else. Her consideration for others' feelings was sabotaging her own needs.

If an Empathetic Eater plans a healthy dinner but her kids demand chicken nuggets, she gives in. When her friend gets dumped and wants to get drinks for three nights in a row, she can't say no. She even gives up her evening walk plans to watch TV with her husband because he wants her to.

While blaming the inability to meet your goals because you are catering to others is socially acceptable, it will keep you stuck. Continuing to neglect your physical and mental wellbeing in the name of service also leads to resentment and can negatively impact your relationships.

Stick up for yourself. Just because someone wants you to split loaded nachos and a pitcher of beer doesn't mean you have to (unless, of course, you want to!)

Food Mood and Body Journal

After we finished completing one week of meal planning, it was time to implement a healthy form of tracking Claire's progress. Monitoring how she felt during her journey was necessary for staying on track for the long haul.

"Taking time to reflect on *why* you eat is just as important as considering what you're eating," I told Claire. "Traditional food tracking applications that emphasize counting calories and weighing food don't encourage self-reflection or listening to your body. A sustainable approach to healthy living requires mindfulness around food and how your habits impact your physical, mental, and emotional wellbeing. That's where keeping a *Food, Mood, and Body Journal* comes in handy."

"Okay... so you don't want me to count calories or track macros?"

"Nope," was all I said back, wondering why Claire sounded disappointed. Didn't she want a break from the obsessive tracking? Didn't she want to stop feeling like a caged lab rat being fed nothing but dry pellets and oats on a strict time schedule? I was about to set her free to eat, well, whatever it is wild and healthy critters enjoy!

Resting her chin on the back of folded hands, Claire set her elbows on my desk. She squinted her eyes at me. I squinted back. After a moment, she murmured, "What if I don't trust my body to tell me how to eat without a calorie count?"

It wasn't disappointment she felt. It was fear.

"You can learn," I enthused, "with a *Food, Mood, and Body Journal.*"

"A what?"

"A *Food, Mood, and Body Journal*. It's a food log that provides space for you to record not only *what* you eat, but *when, where*, and with *whom*."

"Sounds like detective work," Claire said.

She wasn't wrong! Keeping a food journal allows Food Trackers to collect "clues" as to why they make certain choices.

Instead of obsessing over how many calories are in each meal, or if a food is "bad," journaling aids Food Trackers in developing a style of eating that promotes mental and physical wellbeing. They can use the data to make mindful eating decisions and ultimately have a better relationship with their food and body.

By committing to a Food, Mood, and Body Journal, my client Dee discovered she often ate whatever her twin toddlers left on their plates. She didn't even like dino nuggets, but she'd pop half-eaten pieces in her mouth simply because they were in front of her face. With new-found awareness, Dee was able to toss out the leftovers and feel more in control of her choices.

My other client Rebecca discovered she would leave work feeling irritable and hungry. When she got home, she'd open the pantry in a frenzy and snack on whatever she could find. By the time her partner served a healthy dinner, she had no appetite. Her *Food, Mood, and Body Journal* helped her plan a protein-rich snack to eat at the office, so she didn't overdo snack chips or crackers at home.

When I kept my own *Food, Mood, and Body Journal*, I discovered smoothies did not keep me full as long as other breakfast options. I feel much more satisfied eating a solid meal. If I'm craving a smoothie, I drink one as a snack or pair it with something I can chew such as almond butter toast.

"Another difference between Food, Mood, and Body Journals and traditional food tracking apps is the emphasis journaling puts on what to eat more of, rather than what to restrict. We know from studies the more you restrict food, the more you're going to crave it."

"Like in rat studies?"

I laughed as I turned to my laptop and pulled up PubMed, my go-to resource for scholarly articles. "Yes, like rat studies but with sugar! It's been found that rats with restricted access to sugar are more likely to binge than the ones who are offered both unlimited amounts of sugar and regular food."

"When I track food, I do feel restricted," Claire confessed. "I suppose that's why I eat everything I shouldn't on weekends."

"Exactly. Telling yourself you shouldn't eat something means you'll want more."

"This reminds me of Cody, my 8th grade crush," Claire grinned. "I thought he was so cute, but he paid me no mind, so I became *obsessed* with getting his attention. He consumed all of my thoughts! In 10th grade when he finally took notice of me, I realized he wasn't all that."

"We want what we can't have," I replied. "There's a Minnesota Starvation Diet Study where a group of men were put on restrictive diets and subsequently developed obsessions with food and cookbooks. This experiment suggests that extreme dieting negatively impacts an individual's physical, social, behavioral, and psychological well-being."

"Reminds me of my dad, who briefly competed in wrestling tournaments when I was growing up," recalled Claire. "While he followed a strict diet to cut weight, he'd zone out to cooking shows and plan all of the meals he wanted to eat after his competition."

"Let me guess, he'd joyfully stuff his face for days or weeks following his tournament, regaining any of the weight he lost?"

Claire nodded. To keep her from falling into the same cycle, we reviewed the BNT Protocol and discussed the two different methods for keeping an effective *Food, Mood, and Body Journal*.

"You can either freestyle your journal in a notebook, the notepad app on your phone, or use a digital application specifically for mindful food tracking, *not* calorie or macronutrient counting. There are food journals such as a phone app called Ate[13], which allows users to simply snap a picture of their food and reflect on how it made them feel with guided questions about where, why, and with whom they ate. I like this application. It gives you a visual overview of everything you ate, helps set mindfulness goals, and lets you observe the impact of food."

"Sounds interesting, but I am more of a pen-to-paper gal," Claire admitted. "I like to spend as much time off my phone as possible. How would you recommend I keep a journal in a notebook?"

To keep things simple and effective, I recommended Claire keep track of just five data points: what she ate, when she ate, where she ate, how she felt before eating, and *how* she felt after eating.

At the beginning of each day, I wanted her to journal one line about her ultimate health goals and intentions around food such as meal planning, eating per the BNT Protocol when she was hungry, or being kind to her body. This would serve as a reminder of her ultimate health goals and keep her on the right path. At the end of each meal or day, Claire could also add any relevant notes or observations to her food journal.

I showed Claire an example of a *Food, Mood, and Body Journal*:

---

[13] *Learn more about Ate app at https://youate.com/. I have no affiliation with the application- just an avid user!*

Daily Intention: *Follow the BNT Protocol*

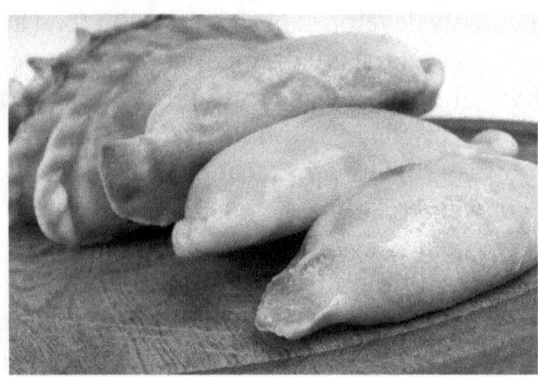

What: *2 beef and cheese empanadas*

When: *12:30 pm*

Where: *Local Colombian cafe*

Before eating, I felt: *Ravenous*

After eating, I felt: *Uncomfortably full, sleepy*

Notes: *Began to feel hungry at 11 AM but felt like that was too early to eat lunch. Waiting to fuel led to a snap decision and overeating. Next time, I'll eat when I feel hungry and order just one empanada that includes vegetables.*

"This seems doable," Claire said as her eyes scanned my example. "But I have a few questions. What if my daily intention is the same every day?"

"Great," I replied. "Repetition builds habits."

"Do I have to journal everything I eat at the time I eat it?"

"Nope, that's not always realistic. You can do it all at once, either the night of, during a lunch break, or the next morning," I said, adding it was OK if she missed a few meals or if some of her entries were less complete than others. "As long as you touch base with your *Food, Mood, and Body Journal* at least once per day for a minimum of 60 days, you'll be on your way to reaching your goals."

"What if life happens and I miss a day?" Claire asked.

"It's not a diet, so don't wait until the following Monday to restart," I said. "Pick it up again the following morning and keep going until you have a total of 60 food logs, even if they're not consecutive."

A food journal doesn't need to be perfect to work. It just needs to be done.

Your Turn

Either digitally or on paper, begin keeping your own *Food, Mood, and Body Journal* for at least 60 days. If using a digital method, I recommend The Ate App on your smartphone. If using a tangible journal, answer the following prompts to get your started.

- *Daily Intention:*

- *What I Ate:*

- *When I Ate:*

- *Where I Ate:*

- *Before Eating, I felt:*

- *After Eating, I felt:*

- *Notes:*

Factory Settings

Anyone can meet with a dietitian for an hour, but it takes an intentional individual to devote themselves to changing their habits. The real magic happens during the mundane moments—getting off the couch to meal plan after a wild Saturday night, choosing to fuel with a substantial meal when snacking chips sounds inviting, getting a pan dirty cooking eggs for breakfast instead of grabbing a sugary bar. Over time, it's these small moments that yield a big change.

As I do with all of my clients, I sent Claire a check-in email a few days after our first session to see how she was doing. Six days had passed, and all I heard were crickets. I was worried she was one of the clients who mistakenly thought paying for a dietitian's services was enough to turn a new leaf. Right as I opened up my phone to shoot her a text, I heard a *ping* from my email application.

A message from Claire. Was she telepathic? I scanned my office for hidden cameras and opened the email. It read:

Hey Kait!

> *Hope you're doing well.*
>
> *I apologize for my delay. Between meal planning, journaling, and the demands of life, I've been neglecting my email inbox.*
>
> *However, the never-ending string of messages has been worth it as I am proud to say I've planned at least 75% of my meals since we last met! Going to the grocery store twice a week and cooking meals at home means I'm eating out way less, which makes me feel like I am making progress.*
>
> *Due to circumstance, there were a few times I was unable to journal or stick to my plan. While I still feel slightly guilty about this, it helps to remember I have the next day planned. This makes it easy for me to focus on the big picture.*
>
> *I'm still working on building confidence around my food choices. There are times when I second-guess whether a food is good or bad, but I am getting better at ignoring them and focusing on eating more nutritious foods per The BNT Protocol.*
>
> *Paradoxically, I haven't been craving as much junk food. Last night at the bowling alley, my teammate brought a box of cereal that was supposed to taste like ice cream. I sampled a little but didn't feel the need to pour a whole*

bowl. I attribute this to eating well throughout the day and not restricting myself from enjoying sugar.

I must confess something to you. Last week, I told my mom I was working with you. She laughed and said I didn't need a dietitian to lose weight, I just needed to eat less than 1200 calories a day. Feeling anxious, I tracked my food into a calorie counter for an entire weekend. As I was doing it, I realized how miserable meal tracking made me. I deleted the app and kept true to the goals we set.

I haven't weighed myself, but I know I am changing both mentally and physically. For the first time in a long time, I feel confident I can stick to something for the long haul. I'm excited to see where this leads!

See you next week,
Claire

A common mistake Food Trackers make is believing as soon as they quit dieting and start fueling their body, they'll completely transform within weeks and never struggle with food again. If only this were true!

In reality, breaking disordered eating habits takes time, which can be very frustrating to the women who are used to quick fixes. There will be days where Food Trackers lapse back into old habits, or as my therapist calls them, factory settings.

Factory Settings are default behaviors or thought patterns a person has had for years. It's normal to fall back on them when we feel triggered or don't see results as quickly as we'd like.

Chantel, a former Food Tracker and client, reverted to her factory settings of obsessively weighing herself the moment she felt bloated before starting her period. Once she decided to throw her scale out, she was able to accept the natural shifts in weight that occur during her cycle. Instead of dieting, she focused on fueling with filling foods and staying hydrated.

In Claire's case, she fell back into her factory setting of calorie counting when her mom made triggering comments about her new way of thinking. Within two days, Claire realized her factory settings weren't going to get her to her ultimate goal and ditched the food tracking.

Other examples of unhealthy Factory Settings with food include:

- Eliminating or reducing entire food groups or macronutrient groups

- Stepping on the scale throughout the day

- Weighing food, including in inappropriate settings such as restaurants

- Body checking[14]

- Skipping meals to save calories or "make-up" for food eaten prior

- Juice cleansing or detoxing to lose weight quickly before events

Recovering Food Trackers must recognize patience is a virtue and the occasional set back is **not** a failure! In fact, it's a universal experience for any All-or-Nothing Dieter hoping to make lasting changes. By keeping a *Food, Mood, and Body Journal,* dieters can stay focused on their ultimate goals and rewire their Factory Settings to benefit their wellbeing.

Your Turn

List any of your unhealthy Factory Settings.

Consider your ultimate health goals. Which healthy behaviors can you replace these Factory Settings with?

As we worked together for the next six weeks, Claire discovered she slipped into her Factory Settings less and less. However, the urge to weigh her food or count calories didn't go away completely. Although less influenced by her mother's judgmental comments about food and

---

[14] *Body checking is continuously seeking information about one's weight, size, or appearance. It interferes with focus and daily routines, and negatively impacts self-esteem.*

her weight, Claire had to continuously remind herself her journey was unique to her and *only* her.

"I can't change my mom, but I can change how I respond," she told me at one of our final sessions. I noticed Claire no longer hid her body dressed in baggy sweats. She wore a fitted T-shirts and breezy gym shorts. I took this as a subtle sign she felt more comfortable in her body.

"Speaking of your mom, how are you feeling about the Lunar New Year?"

"Walking into family functions always feels like entering battle, but this time I am armed and ready." Claire sat a little upright as she spoke and flipped her long braid. "Understanding my mom is from a different generation and was a victim of diet culture herself has not only allowed me to empathize with her, it's given me permission to react differently to her comments about my weight and body."

"How so?"

"For one, I realized calorie counting and following plans like *Fat to Fit* only felt like solutions but in reality, they made me feel worse about my body. When my mom suggests them, I have to remember she doesn't know what's best for me when it comes to my health and accept she's not willing to learn. She's still a great mom and I love her, but taking care of my body and self-esteem means ignoring her comments."

I nodded in agreement. Although Claire would encounter more battles with food and body image throughout her journey, she was on the right track to healing generational trauma. If Claire became a mother, the shame around weight and food would end with her.

"Has daily journaling helped you build more trust between you and your body?"

Claire nodded. "Totally. It's a place for me to vent when I'm triggered and return home to my body. As a result, I'm feeling better throughout the day without obsessing over how many calories I have left for dinner. It's strange because I thought recording every morsel of food would make me feel at ease about eating, but it's clear tracking made me feel *more* anxious. I've deleted the calorie counting app, and I'm never getting it back."

Shadow Integration:

- Recognize why you diet or where your beliefs about "good" and "bad" foods started. Then, practice self-compassion and forgiveness. You or your family thought dieting was the best solution, and you were only trying to do what you thought was best at the time.

- Leverage desire for structure and organization by planning your meals and fitness goals ahead of time.

- To help you become mindful about your eating habits, replace calorie or macronutrient counters with a Food, Mood, and Body Journal.

- Instead of measuring your progress with your weight, track changes in your energy, mood, fitness, or confidence.

Chapter Takeaways:

- Create a vision for your ultimate health goals, including how you want to look and feel around food. Use this vision to help you throughout the book!

- Reflect on how your parents' views on food and body image influence your thoughts

- Labeling foods as "good" or "bad" is an unhelpful strategy that creates fear around eating

- Stop waiting until Monday to "start over"

- Meal planning can provide structure for what to eat and keep you focused. Follow The 5 Steps to Meal Planning to get started!

- Practice meal planning until it's a habit

- Tune into your natural hunger cues and response to foods by keeping a *Food, Mood, and Body Journal* for at least 60 days

- Factory Settings are default behaviors and thought patterns that keep you stuck in old habits

Chapter 2
The Perfectionist

Shadow Tendencies:

- Self-critical

- Rarely feels satisfied with positive results

- Seeks approval and acceptance of others

- Prioritizes other opinions before her own

- Criticizes other eating behaviors or bodies

- Struggles with vulnerability

- Commonly experiences digestive issues related to Irritable Bowel Syndrome (IBS)

The Perfect Diet Does Not Exist

After being adopted from Russia when she was a one-year-old, Mila spent the last four decades of her existence trying to fit in…

A Ted Baker size 4 dress.

With her mother and sister, who were biologically related.

A culture that wanted her to stay small when all she wanted was to take up space.

Now, she came into my office with the goal to fit back into the "normal" Body Mass Index (BMI).

"My BMI is 26.2, putting me in the overweight range by 1.3 points," Mila told me with a sense of urgency in voice. "According to this chart, I must lose at least five pounds to get back down within the normal range. I'd like to lose an additional five pounds so I never slip back into being overweight again."

Mila flipped her iPhone screen towards me to display an outdated BMI chart.

I used my fingers to zoom into the image. "While it may feel jarring to be labeled as overweight, your BMI doesn't define you or your health," I gently explained. "It's based on an outdated formula made up by a 19th century mathematician, not a physician. It only compares your height and weight, but doesn't account for other factors such as your muscle mass, waist-to-hip ratio, or bone density. A shredded bodybuilder with less than 10% body fat can be categorized as overweight, even obese, based on BMI."

I tried not to feel offended as I watched Mila pull out a disinfecting cloth from her bag and wipe the screen I barely touched. In fact, everything about Mila screamed *sterile*. She wore a neatly pressed pink tennis skirt and stain-free white polo with equally clean Asics. Despite coming from practice, not one of her shiny strawberry blonde hairs were out of place in her slicked back pony tail. When Mila spoke, not a single crease on her forehead or around her eyes surfaced. There were no blemishes on her chiseled jawline, clumps of mascara in her lashes, or chips in her nail polish. The woman was flawless, and I'll admit it was hard for me to believe someone so put together would recruit the help of someone as imperfect as me. I suddenly felt a bit insecure about my dry, split ends and slightly crooked teeth.

Although Mila was noticeably tall with wider hips and broad shoulders, by no means did she appear overweight. In fact, the muscle tone in her arms and calves made it obvious she spent plenty of time in the weight room or on the tennis court.

"I still don't like it," Mila replied with a flat tone, referring to her BMI. "It doesn't feel good to hear from your physician that you are classified as overweight, especially when I do so much to stay healthy."

I empathized with Mila. Even if she had conscious awareness that her BMI didn't define her, I understood how being flagged on a medical chart could feel like a loss. Many of us women were brought up to believe being overweight meant we were less lovable or worthy in the eyes of others. This simply is not true. It's our character, our hearts, and how we treat others that should define us, not our bodies. It takes a lot of patience and inner work to reprogram deep-rooted beliefs and comments from doctors, loved ones, and internet trolls, all of which keep us stuck in negative self-talk loops.

"If the BMI did not exist and you were never told you were overweight, how would you feel about *your* body?" I asked Mila.

"I believe I'd still try to lose weight," she said, pinching the skin of her thigh. "I just don't feel comfortable in my body."

"When *was* the last time you felt comfortable in your body?"

"Perhaps around the time I finished primary school, age 11 or 12."

Any flicker of expression on Mila's face vanished as quickly as it appeared. I waited for her to go on, but she just stared back at me.

"So... puberty?" I finally asked, breaking the thick silence between us.

Mila nodded, refusing to go into more detail. I realized I needed to approach Mila differently than other clients, many of which are open books and break down into tears within the first five minutes of our meeting. In order for Mila to trust me and listen to any recommendations, I couldn't push her out of her emotional comfort zone too quickly. Rather than ask her to go into detail about her relationship with food during adolescence, I went with something a bit more surface level.

"Puberty was a long time ago. You have a completely different body as a grown woman. In fact, I'm guessing your body has changed several times over the years. Now that you're in your 40's, does being comfortable in your body mean something different than it did when you were 11, 18, or 30?"

"Interesting question." Mila paused to think. "It's the same in that I've never felt like I've reached my full potential with how I look. No matter what age, I've always felt like I could be slimmer. At age 11, I was comparing my body to my classmates and sister. When I was 21, it was easy to replace a few meals with shakes and lose a few pounds. Around age 32, I noticed a shift. I wasn't able to drop weight after trips or vacations, and it made me frantic. I've always been afraid of getting fat."

She shifted in her seat as her eyes glanced around the room. Was she judging the decor? Or the stack of vintage nutrition books my colleague collected, including one titled *Constipation?* I'd figured out talking about her feelings didn't come naturally to Mila, so I was proud she had mustered the courage to be vulnerable. I posed a hypothetical situation to see if she'd open up more.

"Let's say you did lose five to ten pounds to fit within the normal range of BMI. Do you think you'd feel comfortable then, or would the voice in your head telling you to be thinner continue?"

"I...I'm not quite sure," she stated, looking up as though the right words were tucked behind the ceiling tiles. "I'd like to say I'd be content, but I think I'd still be unhappy. Even at my fittest, I've never felt satisfied. I look back at old pictures of myself and think I look fantastic, though I can distinctly remember feeling chubby when the photo was taken."

"It sounds like you haven't accepted anything less than perfect."

"You could say that."

"Being perfect is a lot of pressure to put on yourself, huh?"

"Ha! I'm used to pressure." Mila clapped her hands and leaned back. "In fact, I thrive under pressure. Always have, thanks to Mother."

Now we were getting somewhere.

"Did your mother expect you to look perfect, too?"

"If she did, she never let me know," Mila scoffed. "She rarely complimented me, despite me trying everything in my power to gain her approval. Unlike my sister Mischa, I was adopted and looked nothing like the women in my family. They were naturally petite whereas I am not and never will be. In fact, I think I startled Mother when I hit puberty before Mischa, who is eighteen months older. My large bone structure and tall stature made me feel like an outsider in my class and at home."

"That must have been hard," I replied, thinking back to my own experience in school. I remembered having to line up by height in 5th grade gym class. I was always the tallest girl and thought it was awesome until the class bully told me boys preferred short girls. Suddenly ashamed, I would bend my knees in class photos to keep from feeling like a giant next to my smaller classmates.

"It didn't kill me," Mila shrugged, still expressionless. "Mother was a tough lady, and she rarely said anything complimentary to anyone. Well, except Mischa."

"Did your mother and sister's eating habits influence yours?"

Mila cackled. "Oh, Mother would have *loved* that."

"What do you mean?"

"Mother never said anything, but I knew she didn't approve of my eating habits. She'd give me this look and shake her head whenever I asked for a second serving at dinner or when she caught me snacking between tennis practice and piano lessons." Mila paused and pursed her lips. "Compared to her birdseed diet, any amount of food looked like a lot. Mother would only eat buttered toast and coffee for breakfast, a half sandwich and tea for lunch, and a toddler-sized portion for dinner. I rarely saw her indulge in desserts, even though she baked for my father and brother on a weekly basis."

Wow, I thought. *If I'm taking the time to bake brownies, I'm claiming half the pan for myself.*

"So your mother wanted you to eat, er—*not eat*—like her, but she wouldn't directly address the topic of food with you." I thought about Claire whose mother made comments about her eating habits at the table. "Instead, she gave you judgmental glances and praised your sister?"

"Right." Mila smiled softly but had a sad look in her eyes. "I still feel this immense pressure to be perfect and make Mother happy, just as my sister naturally did. I tried so hard to live up to her standards. I played piano, did ballet, and got straight A's, but I know she was embarrassed by my weight."

"Did she ever tell you that?"

"She didn't need to. It was evident in how she treated me versus Mischa, who was thin and beautiful."

Mila's fear of gaining weight began early in childhood. She associated living in a larger body than her mother as being imperfect, which in her mind was synonymous with being unlovable. And who could blame her for feeling this way? Her mother, the person she needed unconditional love and acceptance from, made Mila feel lesser compared to her sister Mischa. Regardless of whether her mother actually treated Mischa better because of her appearance, Mila's childhood self made the association that *perfection* would earn her love. She's been chasing it ever since.

Your Turn

Answer the following questions. Do you…

- Criticize yourself?

- Criticize others?

- Wish to be thinner or fitter, regardless of your weight?

- Crave approval from others?

- Get defensive when receiving constructive feedback?

- Procrastinate goals, deadlines, or tasks on your to-do list?

- Rarely feel satisfied with yourself, your work, or your projects?

- Have trouble moving past mistakes, no matter how big or small?

If you answered "yes" to three or more of these questions, you may identify with the shadow tendencies of The Perfectionist sub-archetype. The strategies in this chapter will help you manage your perfectionist tendencies around food and eating.

Peanut Butter Breath

"How did your mom's unrealistic expectations impact your relationship with eating?" I asked Mila.

"I certainly developed a preoccupation around food," Mila continued. "Since Mother packed me a tasteless lunch, I'd trade school supplies for my classmates' snack cakes. I can't believe I'm telling you this, but I'd scarf them in the locker room before tennis practice so there was no evidence."

I was pleasantly surprised by Mila's vulnerability. It can take a few sessions for some Perfectionists to admit any food-related secrets aloud.

"You were growing, hungry, and didn't feel safe to eat at home without getting judged," I commented. "I don't blame you for running a trading scheme. I would have, too."

Mila paused before speaking. "I never would have used the word *unsafe*, but that is how I felt. I'll never forget the time Mother caught me sneaking peanut butter by the spoonful in the pantry. I tried to hide the jar behind my back so she wouldn't see, but I was busted. Without a word, she snatched the jar, placed it on the top shelf, and looked at me like I was a disgrace. From then on, she'd periodically ask to sniff my breath when I walked out of the kitchen to see if she could smell peanut butter. I only dared do it when she was not home."

I actively had to keep my jaw from dropping. I've heard a lot of stories from clients about their parents' warped relationships with food, but none where a parent was smelling the breath of their child to catch them eating peanut butter!

"That must have been so stressful," I said. Stressful felt like the wrong word… It was traumatizing? Clinically insane?

"It was. In fact, I still sneak eat," she admitted. "I keep a secret stash of gelato in our garage freezer, and it's not uncommon for me to have a big bowl as soon as my husband leaves for work at 9 AM. I don't want him to see me eating bad food, especially when he knows I'm trying to lose weight."

"I know you judge yourself for eating gelato, but do you think your husband would really care?"

"No, not at all," Mila said, revealing a half smile for the first time since meeting me. "He could care less about nutrition, really. The man has zero food complexes."

I assumed by the term *food complex,* Mila meant her husband had no unhealthy beliefs around food and eating. He ate to live, enjoying delicious flavors without fearing whether a buttery dinner roll would affect his weight or sense of self-worth.

"What does he think of your BMI? Or that you're seeing a dietitian to lose weight?"

"He always tells me I don't need to lose weight, and he likes me for exactly how I am," she said, her face softening for a moment. "He supported me when I told him I was going to see a professional."

"He sounds like a non-judgmental gem," I said. "So why hide the ice cream from him?"

Mila looked down, fiddling with a stunning emerald cut diamond ring on her finger. Its elegance and class suited Mila perfectly.

After a moment, she deflected my question by explaining how she successfully kicked the gelato habit by following a 30-day sugar detox challenge. "I can abstain from sugar the whole month, but I inevitably revert to my old ways once the thirty days are complete."

Instead of healing her core wounds around perfectionism, Mila slapped a Band-Aid on her sneak eating and was surprised when it didn't resolve her pain. Diets disguised as 'detox challenges' gave her a brief sense of control, then convinced her *she* was the problem when she couldn't make an unsustainable approach stick.

For Mila, dieting reinforced a core belief that no matter how hard she tried, she would never be *good enough*.

"When I was younger, I believed I needed to be thin to be loved or attractive," I shared with Mila. "To maintain an unrealistically low body weight, I dieted *hard*. Like you, I was afraid gaining weight would make me a reject. It wasn't until I recognized how this core belief was untrue and actually fueled my eating disorder."

The look in Mila's piercing eyes suggested she was surprised her dietitian was admitting to body image and eating struggles.

I continued, "Once I decided that I was lovable and worthy no matter what I looked like, I was able to focus on eating to feel good. For me, this was following The BNT Protocol 80% of the time. I stopped trying to look and be perfect. Now, I feel more confident in my skin than ever! Plus, I have a partner and a wide circle of friends who love me at any and every size."

Your Turn

Which core beliefs make you feel like you need to diet, lose weight, and/or look perfect? Core beliefs I've seen in Perfectionists include needing to look perfect or thin to be liked; never feeling good enough at any weight or size; and needing to eat cleaner (or stricter, or healthier) to be worthy.

How are these core beliefs influencing your eating and health habits?

How about your mental health?

Hunger Does Not Equal Failure

The first step to helping Mila stop sneak eating was to teach her The BNT Protocol. Because Mila was restricting her portions at meals, she also needed to understand how to regulate her hunger and satiety cues. However, daily hunger levels are unpredictable, which is a tough reality for some Perfectionists to accept.

"As much as I wish it were possible to feel satisfied eating the same portions of the same foods at the same times each day, the human body is not wired for strict eating schedules," I explained to Mila. "Some days you'll be hungrier than others. That's normal and completely healthy."

The statement is especially true for women who menstruate. Our bodies run on a 21-40 day cycle. Hormonal shifts explain why we may feel like a bottomless pit right before our period but have a lower appetite the following week. Or why we crave cheesecake with a side of potato chips once a month, but find it to be an unappetizing combination other days. Hormonal shifts during our cycle also explain why some women feel motivated to train for a 5k during their follicular phases[15] but can only muster up the energy for a slow walk during their luteal phase[16].

On the other hand, men's bodies run on 24-hour hormonal cycles. This makes it easier for them to repeat the same workouts and meals day after day. While they're not totally immune to fluctuations in appetite, they collectively experience less fluctuations in energy and cravings. All to say, if a man judges you for eating or resting more before your period, you have my permission to school him.

Perfectionists often have trouble trusting their bodies to self-regulate. This stems from developing disordered eating habits as adolescents, comparing their own eating habits to the habits of others, and most common, following strict diets. The longer they try to control every variable around eating, the more they disconnect from their intuitive knowledge about how much and what to eat.

In order to regain trust with their appetite regulation, Perfectionists must relinquish *some* control over what they eat. This doesn't mean throwing caution to the wind and stuffing their faces with bonbons all day. It's putting an end to micromanaging food and seeking a healthy middle ground instead. This middle ground provides a level of safety while allowing Perfectionists to reconnect with their body's intrinsic cues including appetite, cravings, and preferences.

---

[15] *The follicular phase refers to the first half of a menstrual cycle, following the period. Estrogen levels begin to rise, resulting in a spike in energy and mood. Many women feel most productive and motivated during this time!*

[16] *The luteal phase follows after ovulation, typically lasting 14-16 days. Estrogen lowers and progesterone increases, which may lead to a drop in mood and energy. It's a great time to slow down, rest, and incorporate lower impact movement.*

The Hunger Scale:

For women who struggle with understanding hunger cues, I recommend using a Hunger Scale, adapted from the Intuitive Eating™ approach to eating.

The Hunger Scale is a tool used to better understand varying levels of hunger and fullness and how to respond to each sensation. From 1-10, each number represents physical and mental sensations associated with a level of hunger or fullness. Refer to the Hunger Scale before and after meals, and record your ranking in your food, mood, and body journal.

1- Painfully Hungry: So starved you feel dizzy and lightheaded, sometimes with an upset stomach or nausea.

2- Hangry: Feeling moody, irritable, and distracted by the empty pit feeling in your gut that won't go away.

3- Hungry: Thoughts of food become frequent as your stomach rumbles; you feel like you need energy.

4- Somewhat Hungry: Stomach feels slightly empty but hunger doesn't feel urgent. You may think, "I could eat."

5- Neutral: Neither hungry or full.

6- Somewhat Full: Stomach feels full but not completely satisfied. Thoughts of food become less intense or frequent.

7- Satisfied: Stomach feels comfortably full, and you're ready to move on to your next task.

8- Too Full: You feel full, slightly past the point of comfort. You may feel the need to rest and digest before moving on to your next task.

9- Uncomfortably Full: Stuffed to the point of needing to change into loose fitting clothing. You may want to take a nap.

10- Binge: Physical discomfort to the point of feeling sick or nauseous, often follows a binge eating episode.

Your goal is to eat when you feel between a 3 or 4 and stop when you feel like 7. Waiting to eat once you drop to 1 or 2 leads to cravings and overeating to an 8, 9, or 10!

Perfectionism & People-Pleasing

Once Mila understood the fundamentals of balanced eating and appetite regulation, the next step required her to collect evidence that proved her core belief of not being good enough was false. To do so, she needed to quit people-pleasing and start showing up as her authentic self.

"Right now, you believe you must appear perfect to gain the acceptance of others," I told her. "As a result, you deny yourself your own dietary wants and needs by restricting your food in front of others. You look like you have it all together but deep down, you feel out of control."

"My sneak eating makes me feel like a phony," Mila admitted, hanging her head. "When I am out with friends, I pretend I am full from eating half of a chicken salad even when I'm still hungry. I'll pretend like I am too full for dessert just to go home and shovel sweets into my mouth."

"There's a difference between ordering the salad and skipping dessert because that is what *you* wanted versus eating it because it fits the image you're trying to project to others," I said. "Eating until you're full and honoring your appetite means honoring yourself above all else. Right now, you're honoring your made-up opinions of others."

Even though decades had gone by, Mila was repeating the same pattern her mother had reinforced in childhood: appear perfect to avoid the pain of disapproval.

On some level, Mila still believed pretending to have a small appetite and a distaste for sugar would shield her from rejection and judgment from present day friends and family. If for some unlikely reason that were true, it meant Mila was rejecting her own needs to manipulate others into admiring an unauthentic version of her.

And *that* is what kept her in a cycle of sneak eating.

Your Turn

Do you eat differently in front of others than you do behind closed doors?

If so....

- Why?

- Do you believe being perfect will earn you the acceptance or adoration of others?

- What would happen if you chose to eat balanced foods in front of your friends and family?

For Perfectionists, gaining weight or eating outside of the restrictions of their diet in front of others is as vulnerable as showing up to a birthday party in their underwear. They feel exposed and terrified of criticism.

While walking into a social event naked is probably not a good idea, being vulnerable around food is! Not only does this give Perfectionists the freedom to be human, they will see who loves them for who they are (and not who they pretend to be).

In fact, most people will want to be around them *more* when they are raw and vulnerable.

"When you honor your hunger and dietary preferences, you give other people permission to do the same," I explained.

"What do you mean?" Mila asked.

"Let's say you really want the egg sandwich at brunch because it's delicious, but you're afraid to order it because you think it's too fattening or has too many carbs," I explained. "Even though the egg sandwich is balanced, you reluctantly order the green smoothie. If you have any friends who are insecure about their own bodies, they may feel pressure to do the same. This is especially true if you make comments about how satiating the smoothie is or how you only eat plant-based foods."

"I hate to admit it, but posing as a health nut makes me feel superior," Mila confessed. "I know that sounds messed up, but I like pretending I don't have issues with food or my body image."

When you grow up being judged for enjoying food, vulnerability is scary, I thought. Her admission made me think of when I lived in my sorority house during the peak of my restrictive dieting years. Every day, the chef offered pizza as a lunch option in case we didn't like the menu's main entree. While other girls enjoyed a couple of slices guilt-free, I ate boring romaine lettuce salads while lying about how pizza was too greasy for me. What a load of shit! I loved pizza, but I pretended I didn't so no one would suspect it was me leaving empty pizza boxes in the trash after a late-night binge. I was like a bank robber denying involvement without even being asked.

If I had just eaten an occasional slice of pizza like a normal person, I wouldn't have over-eaten in secret. But I was studying nutrition, and I mistakenly believed I needed to uphold the image of *Health Nut*.

"I never considered how my strict eating choices may influence my friends' decisions," Mila went on. "I wouldn't care if they ordered French toast for brunch but after hearing me ramble on about my sugar detox, they may have felt uncomfortable ordering anything I deemed as *off-limits*."

"Imagine if you *did* order and finish the egg sandwich," I said. "The only thing your true friends will notice is your relaxed attitude around food. You'd also be satisfied and less inclined to go home and sneak eat."

Mila considered this for a moment, then said, "I suppose to stop the sneak eating, I must order *off-limit* foods in front of people I normally wouldn't have?"

"Yep," I replied. Mila needed to erase her core belief that she was only good enough when she ate perfectly by eating *imperfectly*.

"Okay," Mila's voice was reluctant, the same as when you instruct a child to tidy up his room before he can play Xbox. "Next time I want gelato, I'll eat it in front of my husband because I'm certain he won't make comments or give me a judgmental glance. Just don't ask me to eat sugar in front of my sister yet. I can't let her know I still struggle with dieting."

I agreed, wondering if Mila's sister would project her own warped beliefs about food onto Mila. When people make negative comments about how someone is eating, it is often because they are insecure about their own relationship to food. Confident people who are secure in their bodies and eating habits hardly notice. If they do, they won't judge or make the other person feel worse.

"I suggest you carry out this experiment silently," I told Mila as she packed up her things to leave. "No need to announce to your husband you're purposefully eating something *off-limits* in front of him. Simply eat the gelato, observe his response, and journal about the experience."

Your Turn

Next time you're eating around others, eat what *you* want and not what you think you should eat to appease them. Eat as much or as little as *you* need to feel satisfied. Journal about the experience. If anyone reacts negatively, consider if they're projecting their own food insecurities on to you.

Perfectionism & Procrastination

Along with People-Pleasing, Perfectionism's other best friend is procrastination. In this case, diets are a form of procrastination. Investing in pre-packaged meal replacements, juice cleanses, and low-carb energy bars trick The Perfectionist into thinking she is on the right track when in reality, she's reinforcing her unhealthy relationship to food. Diets give the illusion that she is making or will make progress, when she's actually wasting time.

When the fad diet inevitably fails, The Perfectionist is back at square one wondering why she's been trying for years but nothing has worked.

Despite having a fear of failure, The Perfectionist continues to set herself up for a loss each time she goes on a restrictive diet. To break the cycle, she must stop procrastinating doing the *inner* work. This is terrifying to a Perfectionist because it means facing her flaws and accepting she is human just like everyone else.

But the idea of being an ordinary human with ordinary needs repulses The Perfectionist, as she believes she **must** be special to earn the love or respect of others. Therefore, she refuses to ask herself the tough questions:

Will I really be fulfilled once I'm two sizes smaller?
Why can't I accept myself until I lose weight?
What emotional void is food and dieting filling?

As The Perfectionist continues to procrastinate her own needs and cater to the perception of others, her self-esteem dwindles. And how has she historically managed self-esteem? By striving for perfection, of course. Talk about a vicious cycle!

Your Turn

Reflection: Do you procrastinate taking real action towards your health goals by going on diets?

Perfectionists procrastinate taking action. They only want to do the inner work when conditions are ideal. For instance, my client Gloria kept telling me she'd join a fitness center when her work load calmed down. Instead of squeezing in walks or doing at-home yoga when she could, she insisted she'd start a formal exercise program when her schedule improved. But as soon as she had time to hit the gym, Gloria had a knack for finding new reasons why it was a bad time—traffic, a birthday trip, or a painful sunburn! By waiting for perfection, Gloria never made any progress.

If you are a perfectionist who procrastinates or people-pleases, you can break the cycle by allowing yourself to be vulnerable about your food and body insecurities, first with yourself and then with others.

In Gloria's case, she had to admit she was too nervous to join a gym because she was afraid of being judged. When I suggested fellow gym patrons were more preoccupied with their own appearance, she clarified: *I'm worried about judging myself. I used to be strong and fit, and I'm afraid of feeling out of shape.*

Once Gloria was vulnerable with herself, she was able to initiate a program that met her needs. Instead of hitting a weight room, she signed up for an at-home beginner's weight program and asked a trustworthy friend to keep her accountable.

There are many examples of food & body vulnerability, including:

- Admitting to yourself you actually enjoy the taste of fried food or sugar

- Telling a friend you skipped a workout because you overslept

- Posting your less-than-aesthetic French toast on Instagram (without following it up with a comment you're going to the gym to burn it off)

- Eating popcorn at the movies when your partner doesn't want any

- Not working out on vacation because you want a break

By definition, vulnerability means *being exposed to the possibility of being attacked or harmed, either physically or emotionally.* While most people aren't going to kick or punch you for being honest about your food insecurities, there is a risk of a friend or family member making a hurtful comment. Like Mila, practice being vulnerable in front of someone you are someone who comes from a place of love and neutrality.

Most of the Perfectionist's bad experiences being vulnerable are self-inflicted. She beats herself up for little mistakes or flaws, then tries to fix them by holding herself to impossible standards. Perfectionists with access to therapy are encouraged to make an appointment with a mental health professional. A good therapist will help them uncover why they need to be perfect, give them tools for showing up in the world as their authentic selves, and support them along the way.

I also recommend Perfectionists learn from the queen of vulnerability, Brené Brown. She has a ton of books, but her Ted Talk *The Power of Vulnerability* is free to stream on YouTube.

Your Turn

1. How can you be vulnerable with yourself about your food and body insecurities?

2. Who is someone in your life you can be vulnerable with about your food and body insecurities? How can you practice showing up as yourself around him/her/them?

Boundaries

Days after our vulnerability chat, I texted Mila asking how eating gelato in front of her husband felt.

Mila replied: *As predicted, he did not make any negative comments besides bickering about how I bought espresso gelato instead of pistachio. I beat myself up the whole time I ate it. On the bright side, I stopped at one serving and haven't sneak eaten since. Funny how off-limit foods become less enticing when they're not so forbidden.*

I noticed a new issue related to my people-pleasing...

Can I come in this Friday to chat about it?

When Mila returned to the office, she shared how her perfectionistic tendencies in her career got in the way of her health goals.

"I work as an online professor at a local university, but also own an Etsy shop," Mila shared. "I think a lot of my struggles with eating arise because I work late into the evening. I get so engrossed with filling customer orders or tending to student emails I forget to eat and drink water. Even though I'll make a healthy dinner, it's late. I find myself sneakily eating junk while I cook because I'm starving."

"Does a part of you feel accomplished if you skip meals to keep working?" I asked earnestly.

"Yes." Mila nodded. "It makes me feel like I have power over my body. Plus, it's hard for me to relax leaving work unfinished. I use my job as an excuse not to eat until later, but I realize that also contributes to secret snacking."

"What would happen if you left those orders and emails for the next day?" I asked.

"Yeah right," Mila scoffed. "And risk getting a poor review on my Etsy shop? Or wake up to strongly worded emails from my frustrated students asking when their tests will be graded? It's easier if I just get it done."

For people-pleasers like Mila, saying *no* can feel as uncomfortable as putting the left shoe on the right foot. This leads them to ignore their own needs while catering to others, and eventual resentment.

Learning to say no is a skill that involves creating *healthy boundaries*. Individuals with healthy boundaries express their needs and don't compromise their values to make others feel comfortable. They can politely say no and accept when other people say no to them. They can order whatever they want off the menu and ask judgmental family members or friends not to make any comments.

The best way to set up healthy boundaries without feeling anxious is to use clear, respectful communication.

4 Methods to Communicate Healthy Boundaries

Method 1: If It's Not a Hell Yes, It's a (Polite) Hell No

It's easy to get caught in a cycle of saying yes to every invitation, opportunity, and request. As a result, Perfectionists find themselves with no time for their own health and wellness. To make progress, they need to learn when to say yes and when to say no.

I have found the best way to determine which requests to accept is by listening to my gut reaction. If I feel excited or energized by an event, it's a *hell yes!* It's also a *hell yes* if it's a favor to a person I care about, a task in service to populations I want to help, or if the opportunity moves me closer to my ultimate goals.

Anything less than a *hell yes* is a *hell no*. If my stomach drops at the idea of participating, or if I hesitate but try to convince myself it's a good idea, it's *hell no*. For Perfectionists, any offer that both bums them out and impedes on their wellness should be a *hell no*. Here are some examples on how to give a respectful Hell No:

"Thanks for the happy hour invite, but I committed to a pilates class."

"Dinner and drinks sound delicious, but I have food at home. I don't want to waste it, so can we meet up another day?"

"Thanks for the invite, but I can't make it. Have fun!"

"Your buffalo chicken dip looks delicious, but I'm saving my appetite for dinner."

"Bottomless brunch sounds fun, but Sunday is my only day to run errands and grocery shop."

"No thanks."

Remember, you don't owe anyone an explanation. If they feel disappointed, that's OK. Their feelings are not your responsibility. (Phew!)

Method 2: Communicate Boundaries Ahead of Time

Perfectionists who crack under pressure must consider communicating their boundaries ahead of time. I recommend doing so in a way that 1) acknowledges the other person's effort, 2) states the need, and 3) offers an alternative solution.

Here are three examples of boundaries my clients use to create space for focusing on their health goals:

Problem: Maggie's boyfriend shows his love by bringing home tempting fast food for dinner, even when she doesn't ask for it or already ate. Not wanting to hurt his feelings, Maggie eats whatever he serves.

Communicated Boundary: *"I appreciate you thinking of me, but it's important for me to stop eating fast food. Why don't we save that money for a date night this weekend?"*

Problem: Marc's husband Carlos expects Marc to curl up on the couch after dinner to binge Netflix and ice cream until bed. Marc knows how Carlos looks forward to relaxing all day, but Marc wants to cut back on sugar and be more active.

Communicated Boundary: *"Spending time with you is my favorite, but the best time for me to exercise is after dinner. I'd love for you to join, but otherwise, I'll be back with a protein shake to watch our shows with you after I am done."*

Problem: Jo wants to reduce how much alcohol she drinks for health reasons, but her family celebrates every occasion with wine. Before she can finish a drink, her father is popping the next bottle and refilling her glass. If she objects, he laughs as if it were a joke and tops her off anyway.

Communicated Boundary: *"Dad, I want us all to have fun but please respect my request when I ask you not to refill my wine glass. I don't want to drink more than one glass tonight. If you fill it up anyway, I'll just pour it out. Save it for yourself!"*

When it comes to Mila, I think of her sister and warn her, "Keep in mind that your own actions hold a mirror to others' habits or behaviors. If you get pushback when communicating a boundary, it's helpful to remember they may be projecting their own insecurities. This is your opportunity to ask questions and encourage them to self-reflect."

Like Jo, whose father ignores her boundaries and continues to pressure her to drink with him, she finally asked, "I'm curious as to why you want me to drink, even after I shared why it's important for me to stop?"

Jo discovered her moderation made her dad fear their relationship would change. Historically, they bonded over tasting new wines and popping bottles of champagne. He was also afraid Jo would think less of him if he continued to drink. Approaching the issue from a place of curiosity and patience rather than blame will maintain the integrity of the relationship and help both parties better understand each other.

Mila's idea for a pre-stated boundary was to update her Etsy shop's customer service page to allow her at least 2 weeks to ship orders and 3 business days to respond to inquiries. In her classroom syllabus, she also included a lunch break and wrote she would not be available for communication outside of stated office hours.

She politely said hell no to incessant emails from clients and students with the following responses: *"Thank you for your patience but due to high demand, I am not accepting new orders until next month. Please check back then!"*

"I appreciate your enthusiasm, but test grades will not be posted for another 48-72 hours."

"I'm sorry you missed me, but office hours are from 9-11 a.m. and 2-5 p.m. I am not available outside those hours."

By creating boundaries with her career, Mila would make time to listen to her body and eat when she needed fuel.

Method 3: Schedule Boundaries

Perfectionists are encouraged to schedule times for healthy eating and exercising in digital calendars or tangible planners, then treat them like doctor's appointments. This way, they don't get overbooked.

My client Kendra would start her work day with her schedule 30-40% full but by noon, it was filled with meetings, calls, and webinars. Despite her best intention, Kendra would skip making a healthy lunch and rely on delivery, even though she worked at home!

The solution was to block out a recurring lunch period on her calendar from 12-12:30 p.m. and several 10-minute breaks for healthy snacks and water. She was able to modify her schedule but taking time to fuel herself made it easier for her to reach her goals.

Method 4: Silence Distractions

Taking time to care for yourself during the day can easily be interrupted by texts and emails from friends, family, clients or employers. Don't be afraid to turn your phone on *Do Not Disturb*, exit out of your work-related applications, silence certain friends or client text messages, and opt-out of Instagram notifications to mitigate distractions.

For more guidance on these concepts, I encourage you to pick up the book *Boundaries: When to Say Yes, How to Say No to Take Control of Your Life* by Dr. Henry Cloud and Dr. John Townsend for more tools.

Your Turn

Method 1: What or who can you say *hell no* to so you have more time to take care of your own health and self-care goals?

Method 2: Where can you communicate your boundaries ahead of time?

Method 3: How can you create structured time around your health and self-care activities?

Method 4: How can you silence distractions to help you stay committed?

Misery Loves Company

After Mila set boundaries around her work life, she needed to translate her boundaries to her personal life.

"My sister Mischa and I meet for lunch every other week, and I'm feeling anxious," Mila admitted. "I usually do the worst sneak eating after meals with her."

"Is it because she is judgmental like your mother?" I asked.

Mila nodded. "Even if I order something balanced like salmon, sweet potato, and broccoli, I'm sure she'll say something like, *I could never eat all that food* or *Good for you for eating so many carbs!* To avoid her passive comments, I stick to a simple soup or salad just to devour everything in my pantry when I get home. I want to eat what I want in front of her, but I'm not sure I can handle her snide remarks."

"Confident people don't make others feel bad for having appetites," I stated. "Do you think by putting you down, she's compensating for her own insecurities around food?"

"Maybe? Probably," she replied, pausing to think for a moment. "Actually, I'm not sure. I've always dismissed her bullying as sisterly competition. She always has to one-up me in everything. My husband thinks she learned that when we were kids. When I was adopted into the family, she probably feared she'd lose the attention or love of our parents. Making me feel beneath her ensured she'd be the favorite child, at least in her mind."

Impressed by her husband's psychoanalysis and curious to know more, I asked, "Does Mischa put you down in other areas in your life, such as your marriage or work?"

Mila laughed as if the answer was obvious.

"As much as I want her to be impressed with my life, she never is. I have a stable relationship and a full life with lots of hobbies, but she only likes to hear about my problems. If I tell her about my tennis match, she'll only be interested in the details if I lose."

Turns out Mischa had been in and out of unfulfilling careers and lost touch with most of her friends after high school graduation. She lived alone in a 3,000 sq foot home that she won in her last divorce settlement and spent most of her time cycling through short-term romances with men she found dull.

Misery loves company, I thought but bit my tongue. "Sounds like she lives in a mansion."

"Her home is as massive as it is remarkable."

"Does she make negative comments about your house?"

"No. I think it's because we both know her house is superior to mine, so she doesn't see the point in ripping mine to shreds," Mila said.

"Would you say Mischa only makes you feel bad about things she is threatened by?"

Mila raised an eyebrow. I elaborated.

"Mischa knows her home is fabulous, so she has nothing to prove. If Mischa felt equally as confident about her body or eating habits, would she be judging you for yours?"

Your Turn

Is there anyone in your life who judges your eating habits? If so, how does it make you feel? Is it possible they are projecting their own insecurities on to you?

On the flip side, do you find yourself inwardly or outwardly criticizing other people's bodies or food? If so, what are you projecting?

Letting Go of Perfectionism

If Mila continued to allow Mischa's comments about food to make her anxious, she'd continue to sneak eat after their biweekly visits. To break the cycle, she needed to:

1. Communicate her boundaries ahead of time.

2. Allow herself to be vulnerable with food around her sister.

3. Set goals to eat a balanced diet rather than a perfect one.

"What would happen if you called your sister before your lunch and asked her not to comment on your diet or body from here on out?" I asked Mila after she agreed to set a boundary with Mischa.

"I'd rather text her," she admitted.

"Let's do that now."

"Are you serious?"

"Dead serious."

Mila stared at me for a couple of beats before pulling out her phone and letting out a laugh that said, *I can't believe I am doing this.*

After a couple of rough drafts, Mila settled on the following message:

Good morning, Mischa. I'm looking forward to our lunch date at Armando's. Before we meet, I want you to know I am working with a registered dietitian and have set specific goals for myself around food. I've realized talking about my diet or body image outside of appointments is triggering and therefore, I'd like to keep those topics off-limits tomorrow. Love you & I hope you understand!

"I feel as though I am going to throw-up," Mila said as she hit send. "I'm not sure I quite like this vulnerability thing."

In case Mischa ignored Mila's request and brought up diet-related topics at lunch, Mila brainstormed a few responses to have ready:

"You know I appreciate your perspective, but I'd rather not talk about my diet today."

"Let's change the subject. Have you talked to cousin Ivan lately?"

"I am not discussing this with you."

"I'm proud of you, but it's not over yet," I said. "When you're at lunch, eat the meal that fits *your* needs. Even if Mischa judges you for eating a healthy carb, trust you'll feel satisfied and not go home to sneak eat."

Together, we reviewed Armando's Italian Kitchen's online menu so Mila could pre-select a balanced & healthy meal. When I asked what she normally ordered, she pointed to the *Insalata di Salmone*- a salmon filet served with toasted Italian bread, romaine lettuce, dried cranberries, goat cheese, sunflower seeds, cherry tomatoes, and a citrus Dijon vinaigrette.

"This is a fantastic choice," I cheered. "There's protein and fat in the salmon, fiber in the cherry tomatoes and seeds, and some carbs with the fruit and bread. Plus, the cheese and dressing adds extra fat for flavor and satiety."

"I thought so!" Mila said enthusiastically. "To save calories, I'll also request the chef to leave off the bread, goat cheese, and sunflower seeds."

Like many Perfectionists, Mila believed *low calorie* was synonymous with *healthy*. As a result, she missed out on nutrient-rich foods. Mila noticed my grimace and asked what was wrong.

"Your salmon salad is certainly more nutritious than the mac and cheese," I replied. "But by removing so many ingredients, you're left with just fish atop leaves. That doesn't sound very satisfying."

"Oh," Mila sounded disappointed. "I thought I was being good."

Uh-oh, her people-pleaser was showing. But I wanted her to feel confident about her own decisions so I retraced my steps.

"I shouldn't speak for you," I said. "Do you think your salad will be satisfying with just the salmon and lettuce?"

"No," Mila scrunched her nose. "Not when you put it that way."

"What if you considered ordering the salad *as is* and stopped eating once you feel like a seven on the hunger scale?"

She agreed, but insisted on omitting the goat cheese because she thought it triggered her Irritable Bowel Syndrome[17]. I wanted to encourage her to make decisions based on *her* preferences and body, so I signaled my approval with a thumbs up.

Your Turn

Practice adding nutritious ingredients incomplete meals and snacks. First, identify which macronutrient(s) are missing: carbohydrates, protein, or dietary fat. Then, brainstorm adding healthy foods to make the meal or snack balanced. Use the lists from the Fundamentals of Balanced Nutrition section for help. The first row has been filled in as an example.

---

[17] *Irritable Bowel Syndrome (IBS) is marked by repeated abdominal pain and changes in bowel movements, including constipation, diarrhea, or both. In my personal practice, I notice my clients who report high levels of stress suffer from IBS more often than my clients who report low levels of stress.*

Meal	Missing Macronutrient(s)	Food(s) to Include
Grilled shrimp lettuce tacos with steamed onions, bell peppers, and sliced avocado	Fat & carbs	Mango salsa and sliced avocado
Oatmeal with berries and a banana		
Cheese stick		
Tuna salad with mayo and pickles		
Sweet potato and rice bowl with diced veggies and olives		
Sliced apple with chocolate chips		

Table 2.2.1

Suggested answers are located at the end of chapter.

Balance is In, Perfectionism is Out

The Perfectionist often measures her self-worth based on her ability to follow the rules of a diet, meet societal expectations, or weigh a certain amount. Like Claire The Food Tracker, she thinks in black and white:

I am *good* if I order water, but I am *bad* if I drink a cocktail.

I am *successful* if I burn 300 calories at the gym, but I am a *failure* if I gain a pound the next day.

I am *thin* if I fit into my jeans from college, and I am *fat* if I can't.

In her mind, there is always something to improve. She thinks, *as soon as I fix my weight, then I will be confident, happy, and worthy of love*.

Any bouts of high self-esteem following a "good" day of eating are short-lived as she quickly returns to hyper-fixating on her body or diet. But chasing perfectionism is counterproductive to feeling good. By failing to reach the unreachable, Perfectionists like Mila reinforce the idea that they are not enough.

Seeking balance grants women permission to eat freely without feeling like they're a failure. Balance leaves room for nuance, error, and self-forgiveness. When they combine a nutritious diet with a weekly pizza night and the occasional mocha from Starbucks, they allow themselves to be both healthy *and* human.

Letting go of perfectionistic tendencies by committing to a balanced approach takes guts, especially when there is an underlying belief that relaxing around food automatically means gaining weight. In reality, a balanced approach to eating helps All-or-Nothing Dieters build the confidence and motivation to commit to a healthy lifestyle for the long haul.

"But what does a balanced approach look like in real time?" Mila asked after we discussed why adopting a flexible approach would help her.

"It's different for everyone," I said. "That's the beauty of it! My ideas of balance may look different than yours, but here are some common scenarios comparing a perfectionistic approach to a balanced one."

I whipped out a table comparing a Perfectionist Approach versus a Balanced.

Perfectionist Approach vs. a Balanced Approach

Scenario	Perfectionist Approach	Balanced Approach
A co-worker surprises the office with cookies	Obsesses about whether or not to eat the cookie based on if it fits her calorie or macronutrient goals. If she does eat it, she feels guilty.	Decides whether or not she actually wants the cookie. If she does, she pairs it with her healthy lunch and doesn't obsess over it later.
Oversleeping and missing a workout class	Feels like a failure and/or tries to "make-up" for missing the workout by restricting calories.	Feels disappointed but doesn't stress out. Instead, she adjusts her alarm to wake up early and prevent missing the class two days in a row.
Eating pasta to the point of an 8 on the hunger scale	Feels ashamed and skips break-fast the following day, resulting in low energy.	Laughs about having a food baby and stops eating. She eats her usual breakfast the next day if she's hungry.
Impromptu dinner at a Tex-Mex restaurant with friends	Feels too preoccupied with food, calories, or macros to fully enjoy her company.	Has fun with her friends and orders what will make her feel satisfied and comfortable.

Table 2.2.2

"Notice in these examples how shedding perfectionism does not mean morphing into a careless slob who compromises quality and preferences," I told Mila. "Balance can and should be both realistic *and* effective. Making balanced choices can challenge you, but it shouldn't depress you."

Your Turn

Think of scenarios where you or someone you know takes a perfectionist approach to healthy living. Brainstorm any perfectionist approaches that are holding you back. Then, rewrite these thoughts to reflect a balanced approach that aligns with your goals.

Scenario	Perfectionist Approach	Balanced Approach
Exercise	If I can't work out for an hour, then I won't work out at all.	A 20-minute workout is better than nothing!

Table 2.2.3

SMART Goal Setting

I used to roll my eyes at professional seminars when presenters recommended setting SMART goals. In my mind, the method was too *by-the-book* to actually be effective. It wasn't until I started working 1:1 with clients that I found SMART goal setting proved useful for All-or-Nothing Dieters.

For those who haven't heard of SMART goals, the acronym stands for **Specific, Measurable, Actionable, Realistic, and Time-Bound**.

SMART GOALS

Specific	Measurable	Actionable	Realistic	Time-Bound
Being clear on your goals makes reaching them more achievable	Helps you know when an action is complete and track your progress	Ensures you have control over the tasks needed to complete the goal	Avoids overwhelm and frustration	Helps you stay motivated for the long haul!

For Perfectionists, the specific, measured, and time-bound components of SMART goals come naturally. The Perfectionist will identify she wants to lose 12 ½ pounds in two months, measure her weight daily, and monitor the timeline. If she loses weight, she calls it a success. If she gains weight or the scale doesn't budge, she interprets it as a failure and vows to simply "eat less" or "move more."

However, any weight loss she happens to see is not sustainable because she doesn't measure her success based on her *actions* and her plan is far from realistic.

Perfectionists mistakenly set goals based on **outcomes** rather than **actions.** Goals based on outcomes include ideal weight, body fat percentage, or dress size. While those are acceptable long-term visions, they do not hold The Perfectionist accountable for taking **action** that will move her forward.

One *cannot* actively choose to lose twelve pounds, but one *can* choose what to eat to increase the likelihood she will. Therefore, she should set **actionable** goals around how to eat and track her progress with what she can control. For instance, replacing a sugary coffee with an unsweetened alternative six days per week is an actionable goal she can fully control. Losing ½ lb a day is not.

Because the well-intentioned Perfectionist is used to setting the bar high, even her actionable goals are often not realistic. Even if it's been two years since she stepped into a gym, she'll set a **DUMB** goal to work out every day for two months. (Uh, good luck!)

DUMB is my acronym for goals that are **Delusional, Unreasonable, Mediocre, or Broad**. DUMB goals like "work out every day" seem great at first but fail because they leave too much room for excuses. Instead of working out every day, The Perfectionist must set a SMART goal around exercise that helps her progress but doesn't make her want to give up. An example would be completing three, 30-minute work-outs in her living room during her work-from-home lunch break.

SMART goals should be based on the outcome you'd like to achieve. The following table shares examples of DUMB goals vs SMART goals based on common ultimate visions.

DUMB Goals vs SMART Goals

Ultimate Vision	DUMB Goals	SMART Goals
Fit into old dress	Eat out less	Replace eating out on weeknights with cooking at home at least four nights per week for one month
Get toned	Lift weights	Strength train with a personal trainer twice per week
Reduce cravings	Eat less sugar	Reduce added sugar intake from an average of 35 grams per day to no more than 10 grams per day, six days a week
Live an active lifestyle	Move more	Walk at least 15 minutes after lunch and dinner on weekdays
Feel energized and refreshed	Drink less alcohol	Moderate alcohol intake from 4-6 glasses per week, no more than two glasses of wine on the weekend

Table 2.2.4

"SMART goals should be challenging without being overwhelming," I told Mila. "By breaking big dreams down into digestible chunks, you can move forward and build confidence in yourself."

"How do I know if my SMART goals will help me?" she asked.

This was a good question. Mila needed to paint the picture of her ultimate outcomes and base her SMART goals off what she'd like to achieve. When Mila first came in, her goal was to lose enough weight to fit within a normal BMI. I asked if that had changed.

"Yes and no," Mila's voice sounded strong, as it always had. "After accepting that BMI doesn't define my health, I'm not concerned about being *thinner*. If my weight never changed, I wouldn't care. But I do want to maintain my current level of health by no longer eating in secret."

Internally, I cheered. Outwardly, I remained calm and asked, "How do you want to feel about food and your body?"

"I want to feel at peace." As she said it, Mila closed her eyes and inhaled deeply through her nose. She held the air at the top for a moment, meditating on her declaration.

When she opened her eyes, they looked like that of a caged tiger, released from her pen into the wild. Her narrow eyes signaled she was out for blood, and I pitied whichever unlucky gazelle crossed her path. Throughout our hours together, I hadn't seen Mila appear anything but calm or slightly irritated, but now she looked… pissed.

"I'm tired of fighting against my hunger for the sake of losing a few pounds. I'm tired of trying to appease Mother and win the approval of my uptight sister. I want to feel like myself. My *real* self. No more performative eating in front of others just so they *think* eating healthy and looking trim comes effortlessly to me, because guess what? It doesn't! Not at all. I've fought with my body every fucking day, and I'm fucking sick of it."

I marveled at her answer. It was raw. It was real. For the first time, Mila was owning her decisions.

After such a powerful and vulnerable outburst, it felt inappropriate to change the subject to something as clinical as SMART goal setting and eating more protein. So instead, we spent the rest of the session cursing diet culture and all of the mental damage caused by unrealistic beauty standards. When I admitted I had given in and gotten botox in my forehead, Mila almost spit out her LaCroix.

"Honey, I could have paid your college tuition with how much I've spent on my face," she laughed. "I'm not sure if I'll stop, but I pretend to be *au naturale*."

We were just two imperfect women bonding over our imperfections, and our imperfect need to disguise them.

As our appointment came to a close, I forced myself to change the subject back to nutrition so I could send Mila on her way with next steps. I asked if she wanted to stay an extra five minutes to set SMART Goals with me or do them between now and our next meeting in two weeks. She opted to stay, so we revised her ultimate vision.

"I still want to quit secret eating, but I'm perfectly fine if my weight stays the same," she said. "To do so, I want a balanced diet for life. No more dieting or pretending to eat clean in front of friends just to sneak eat at home. No more letting work get in the way of my wellness, either. I want to feel confident in my choices and not let them influence my decisions."

From there, Mila set three SMART goals:

1. Eat until she was a 6-7 on the hunger scale at meals, especially when dining out with friends or her sister

2. Make time for balanced lunches and dinners by creating work boundaries and scheduling a meal break within her day

3. Practice balancing meals instead of automatically opting for the "cleanest" or lowest calorie option

Your Turn

Based on your ultimate vision, brainstorm three SMART goals:

> **SMART Goals**
>
> •
>
> •

Celebrating Progress, Not Perfection

Mila e-mailed her updates from lunch with her sister.

Kait,

> *After I sent Mischa the text message in your office, it took her seven hours to reply, but she agreed not to say anything. Although I was suspicious she'd ignore my boundary around discussing food and weight at lunch, I was determined not to people-please and stick to my guns. I was pleasantly surprised. Not only did she honor my request, she suggested we split an appetizer because she heard from a friend the bruschetta was delicious.*

I wonder if she too had been restricting how she ate in fear that I would judge her? Perhaps Mischa witnessing me order what I wanted granted her permission to do the same? I'll never ask because I want to pretend that is the truth.

But wait, there's more! I didn't come home after lunch and sneak eat sugar, even though I did consider how good it would taste. I think allowing myself to eat it without conditions has helped me crave it less.

In the meantime, I've been abiding by my scheduled limits at work, most of the time. There was a busy afternoon when I skipped lunch, but I paid for it with a massive appetite later. I identified myself as a "2" on the hunger scale and found it impossible to stop eating before I felt like a 9.

At first, I felt like a failure. Then I remembered to aim for progress and not perfection. I learned from my mistake the next day and stopped for lunch when it was time, which helped me stop working at 6 p.m. for dinner.

I'm looking forward to a brunch with the girls from my country club this weekend. I already know what I am going to order—a cheese and onion omelet with hash browns and fruit. Yum!

As I read the last line, I smiled. The old Mila would have never ordered hash browns, let alone in front of her friends.

I knew this was only the beginning for Mila, but the journey of overcoming perfectionism with food is not linear. There would be triggers pushing her to slip back into her Factory Settings, such as judgmental comments from peers or getting weighed at the physician's office. But with her newfound awareness, Mila would be able to catch herself falling into old habits and return to the vision of her ultimate outcome. From there, she could reset and get back on the right path.

Shadow Self Integration:

- Aim for progress, not perfection

- Being vulnerable with others allows for deeper friendships and more meaningful interactions

- Taking imperfect action is better than not taking any action at all

- Pay attention to the details, but not for so long you don't move forward

- Have a ultimate vision for your health and set SMART goals that move you forward

Chapter Takeaways

- Perfectionists often struggle with people-pleasing and procrastination.

- There are no such things as being "perfect" or having the perfect diet.

- Using The Hunger Scale can help you navigate portion-control and alleviate guilt around natural appetite cues.

- Setting boundaries allows you to achieve great things without overextending yourself.

- Create SMART goals, not DUMB ones.

- Strive for balance, not perfection.

Suggested Answers to Table 2.2.1

Meal	Missing Macronutrient(s)	Food(s) to Include
Grilled shrimp lettuce tacos with steamed onions and bell peppers	Fat & carbs	Mango salsa and sliced avocado
Oatmeal with berries and a banana	Protein and fat	Natural peanut butter and chia seeds
Cheese stick	Carbohydrates	Large piece of fruit
Tuna salad with mayo and pickles	Carbohydrates	Sprouted grain toast
Sweet potato and rice bowl with diced veggies and olives	Protein	Chickpeas and crumbled goat cheese
Apple slices	Protein and fat	Full-fat Greek yogurt as a dip

Chapter 3
The Emotional Eater

Shadow Tendencies:

- Uses food to escape from uncomfortable thoughts, feelings, or situations

- Mindlessly snacks when stressed or bored

- Eats when not hungry, sometimes at unusual hours

- Treats food as a reward (*i.e., I deserve a pizza*)

- Witnesses a parent, guardian, partner, or close family member emotionally eat

- Celebrates positive feelings or events with food

Are you an Emotional Eater?

Emotional eating is like a codependent relationship. But instead of relying on people to cope with uncomfortable emotions, Emotional Eaters use food.

Emotional eating can start innocently enough with a spoonful of chocolate frosting after your toddler's temper tantrum, munching on chips while anxiously awaiting an important email, or diving into a bowl of mac n' cheese after a particularly stressful workday. As long as these behaviors don't interfere with a person's health and wellbeing, it's completely normal to emotional eat sometimes.

But if food becomes a crutch for uncomfortable feelings on a regular basis, emotional eating can spiral into a full-blown dependence and ruin one's relationship to food and body.

For some, emotional eating can surface for short periods after certain seasons. My client Racquel was never an Emotional Eater until she broke up with her long-term partner. For two weeks, she ate banana bread for dinner and washed it down with half a gallon chocolate milk. As soon as Racquel began to move on, she no longer relied on food for comfort.

For others, emotional eating can linger for years or decades. No matter what the situation—fights with friends, bills, traffic—habitual Emotional Eaters primary method of self-soothing is food. In my practice, I define emotional eating as habitual when it occurs *at least* three times a week for over three months.

It's the habitual **Emotional Eater** who often experiences long-term mental and physical consequences such as:

- Distrust around oneself with food

- Unwanted weight gain

- Increased blood sugar levels, cholesterol, or blood pressure

- Fatigue or low energy

- Digestive issues such as bloating or gas

- Guilt or shame around food

These risks can cause inner conflict within the Emotional Eater. Even if she wants to stop using food to cope, her impulse to eat when she's triggered overrides any willpower she thinks she has. Afterwards, she feels guilty, triggering one of two things: more emotional eating or dieting to "make up" for the calories consumed.

For Emotional Eaters who struggle with their weight or health, breaking this cycle is crucial for making lasting changes.

Your Turn

Answer the following questions: Do you...

1. Eat when you feel upset or depressed?

2. What about when you're lonely? Stressed? Bored?

3. Feel urgent needs to eat, seemingly out of nowhere?

4. Eat at unusual times of the day or night?

5. Crave specific types of foods, such as chocolate, after a tough day?

6. Procrastinate doing certain tasks or work obligations by eating?

7. Feel guilt or shame after eating "bad" or "forbidden" foods like sugar, pasta, bread, or chips?

8. Keep "bad" foods out of the house because you don't trust yourself not to overindulge?

9. Snack when you're not hungry more than twice per week?

10. Obsess about the meals or snacks you already ate, so much so you're distracted from other tasks?

11. Skip meals to save up for food you anticipate eating later that day?

If you answered "yes" to three or more of these questions, you may identify with the shadow tendencies of the Emotional Eater sub-archetype. The strategies in this book will help you lessen how often you use food to cope.

The Root Cause

The good news? None of us were born Emotional Eaters. Habitual emotional eating is a *learned* behavior, meaning it can be reversed. It starts with discovering the root issue of emotional eating, then taking an intentional action to resolve the issues and discover new ways to cope without using food.

When determining the root issue, I encourage my clients to reflect on when their relationship to food took a turn for the worse. Emotional Eaters can think back to their childhood or early adolescence for clues. For my client Emma, it was when she was ten years old and watched her parents go through a messy divorce. Blaming herself, she'd hide in her room and self-soothe with candy while she listened to them fight. Now an adult, she turns to sugar whenever life circumstances are out of her control.

For some women, food became the enemy during adolescence when the pressure of being popular and thin started to creep in. Teen girls restricted food groups and skipped meals in an effort to counteract the natural effects of puberty. But in secret, they'd sneak eat popcorn and Reese's cups while wondering why they were the only ones on Earth who couldn't control themselves around food.

Not every Emotional Eater begins in childhood. Others notice that their relationship with food became problematic later in life. This could be due to a career change, having children, injuries causing them to be more sedentary, or hormonal shifts. Instead of learning how to modify their eating habits to fit a new lifestyle or aging body, they dive head-first into a restrictive diet. Along the way, they forget how to listen to their natural hunger cues and find themselves giving into junk when they're stressed or unmotivated.

Common root causes of emotional eating:

- Discovering at a young age that eating is an escape from uncomfortable feelings

- Witnessing family or friends emotionally eat or diet

- Growing up in an environment where family members spoke negatively about their body

- Yo-yo dieting, resulting in fear around many foods or food groups

- Misinformation about how food is metabolized, usually from social media or fad diets

- Exposure to unrealistic body expectations and diet culture via social media, friends, peers, etc.

Regardless of when or why emotional eating became habitual, too many people refuse to do the deep work of eating a balanced diet and coping with their emotions in proactive ways, usually because they're in a hurry to lose weight. They slap a "diet" on the gaping wound and wonder why they continue to bleed.

This was the case for my client Sarah, an Emotional Eater who desperately wanted to gain control over her eating habits and lose weight.

During our first session, she told me, "I've been going to therapy for years and while I've made a ton of progress, what I can't seem to control are my eating habits…"

Sarah didn't need to tell me she was in therapy; she was the most self-aware person I'd ever met! In fact, she even *looked* like a therapist. Slouching back with her legs crossed and holding a clipboard for note-taking, Sarah sported jet black square-rimmed glasses, and her honey blonde hair was pulled back into a tight low bun. Dressed in an edgy oversized navy blazer and slacks, she sat with her arms crossed to hide her belly. Her tone was flat but had a flicker of warmth, reminding me of the girls from high school who were too cool for homecoming parades and prom. My first impression was Sarah looked like the kind of person who didn't care about what people thought but deep down, she was self-conscious about something. To figure out what, I asked her to tell me more about her lack of control with food.

"I use food to cope," Sarah admitted. "I'm only 5'1" but I'm 30 pounds overweight. I think if I trim down, I'll have confidence and feel better about myself. Then, I'll stop making bad choices."

Like many All-or-Nothing Dieters, Sarah believed if she dieted to gain momentum, she'd feel motivated for life and never slip back into her old ways. This was false. What she needed to do was let go of her expectation of quick weight loss so she could discover the root cause of her emotional eating, quit responding to emotional triggers with food, and practice better coping mechanisms.

Your Turn

When was the first time you remember emotional eating? What was the root cause?

The Apple Doesn't Fall Far

As a single mother of two, Sarah's mom worked overtime to keep things afloat. They lived on a tight budget. To distract Sarah and her brother, she sat them down in front of the TV with bags of chips that ended with -os: Doritos, Fritos, and Cheetos. Whenever Sarah's mom had a rough day, the three of them would pile into the car to get Happy Meals and milkshakes.

"That's probably where I learned about emotional eating," Sarah recalled. She went on to share that each time they would go out to eat, her mom would make derogatory comments about herself and her body. "I have a vivid memory of my mom telling me, *No wonder your father left, I'm a fat pig*. We had just left a Chinese Buffet. I tried to comfort her and tell her she was beautiful, but she shut me down. As an adult, I've noticed that I also call myself names when I overindulge. I just keep them to myself."

My heart sank. "That's awful. Did she ever call *you* names?"

Sarah shook her head. Still, her mom's poor self-image had made a lasting impression.

I asked, "If you could go back in time to ask your mom to change how she spoke about herself, what would you tell her?"

"I'd tell her to stop being so dramatic," Sarah said flatly.

Not the answer I expected. For someone who claimed to eat her feelings, Sarah did a great job of pretending she had none. I wondered if her reluctance to open up intensified her emotional eating habits. Was suppressing her feelings with food easier than facing them?

"Fair," I chuckled, deciding to drop the question and pull out the big guns. "How about this? If you could go back in time, what would you tell your younger self as you heard your mom call herself names?"

"Whoa, that's an intense question for a first date," she laughed.

She wasn't wrong. Picturing and speaking to what many psychotherapists refer to as our *inner child* is as triggering as it is healing. Imagine witnessing an eight-year-old saying she needs to stop eating carbs because she is chubby. You wouldn't pinch her tummy and agree she could shed a few pounds! Instead, you'd give her a loving squeeze, reassure her she was perfect the way she was, and tell her to enjoy pizza and cake with her friends. We must speak to ourselves with the same compassion.

"I'd tell the younger version of me," Sarah finally mustered, "that her mom was doing her best, but sometimes she turned to food because she was hurting and didn't have access to therapy back then. The mean things she said about herself were her way of trying to justify why our family was broken. She blamed herself for our struggles."

Sensing she had more to say, I waited.

"I'd tell my younger self it wasn't my job to be strong for my mom. She was allowed to cry and miss my dad, too."

Your Turn

Answer the following prompts:

- If you had the power to change how your relationship to food or your body was influenced as a child or young adult, what would you change?

> • If you could go back in time, what would you tell the younger version of yourself when she began to have unhealthy thoughts about food or her body?

Identifying Emotions

"Now that you're out of your childhood home, do you feel safe expressing how you feel?" I asked Sarah.

"Sort of?" Sarah cocked her head, her voice trailing off. "When I'm in a bad mood, I try not to complain. I don't want to be a nuisance."

Her mother's inability to regulate her emotions left nine-year-old Sarah feeling like she had to be the strong one in her family. She learned to stuff down in an effort to help her mom calm down. This pattern had manifested into a dysregulated relationship with food.

"What kind of bad mood?"

"I dunno. When I'm feeling sad, I guess?" Sarah replied. "Hey, is this therapy? I thought you were a dietitian!"

To better understand which feelings caused Sarah to spiral into emotional eating, she needed to get more specific. Was her sadness rooted in guilt? Powerlessness? Hopelessness? Once she could pinpoint what's going on internally, she'd be able to determine who or what triggered those feelings. From there, she could design her life to better cope with or avoid these triggers and therefore, not rely so heavily on food.

To help Sarah explore her sadness, I pulled out an Emotional Eater Feelings Chart.

"You can use this chart to develop a broader emotional vocabulary and deepen your understanding of your habits. By clarifying your feelings, you can decide what to do about them," I explained.

Emotional Eater Feelings Chart

Feeling	Expression of Feeling
Angry	Frustrated, critical (of self or others), violated, resentful, jealous, hangry (hunger + anger)
Sadness	Depressed, embarrassed, vulnerable, shameful, guilty, powerless, inferior, inadequate, hopeless, disappointment, worthless, deprived
Loneliness	Abandoned, rejected, isolated, excluded, empty
Stress	Anxious, overwhelmed, insecure, nervous, weak, insignificant, anticipatory (negative)
Boredom	Uninspired, apathetic, dull
Happiness	Celebratory, excited, anticipatory (positive)

Table 2.3.1

Using the chart, Sarah identified frustration, depression, and guilt as the key emotions driving her emotional eating.

"I'm a little hot tempered," Sarah admitted with a smirk when I asked about the frustration. "I often get annoyed with other people, and storm off from the situation upset. Munching on something crunchy feels therapeutic. Almost as if the act of crunching is releasing some of that stress. I also struggle with depression. I'm on medications, but the feelings still creep in. I definitely want comfort food when I'm having a depressive episode."

"Do you feel guilty for emotional eating?"

"Absolutely."

"And is eating a distraction from the discomfort of guilt?"

Sarah let out a half chuckle. "Temporarily. After I finish, I don't feel any better. In fact, I usually feel worse."

Your Turn

Using the Emotional Eater Feelings Chart, list which emotions you find yourself consistently numbing with food.

Emotional Eating Triggers

Next, we needed to identify Sarah's *emotional eating triggers*. Emotional eating triggers can include people, environments, or situations that make you want to numb your feelings with food. Triggers can be positive, negative, or neutral.

Below are different situational triggers and examples.

Common Interpersonal Triggers:

- Relatives

- Friends

- Romantic partner

- Romantic partner's ex

- Colleagues

- Roommates

- Social media influencers

- Strangers online

As a client example, Dana had her younger sister Tess move in with her while going to college. As a child, Dana felt insignificant and ugly around Tess who was a naturally lean soccer superstar. When Tess received all of the attention from their parents, Dana felt like a loser but found solace in sugar.

Once Dana left the house after graduation, Dana blossomed. Not only did she land a spot in a competitive internship, Dana also was elected as a representative in Student Government. As her self-confidence increased, her emotional snacking habits slowed down. But within one week of Tess moving in, Dana experienced the familiar feeling of being *less than*. She spiraled back into the emotional eating habits she cultivated as a teen and found herself decompressing with sour gummy worms.

Common Environmental Triggers:

- Workplace

- Kitchens

- Family member's house

- Friend's house

- Childhood home

- Vacation spots or recreational spaces

Emotional eating is not always triggered by unpleasantries. As a personal example, I feel nostalgic and excited whenever I go to the movie theater and smell the buttery popcorn. Snacking during a film enhances the fun of the experience, making it hard to pass up a nostalgic treat.

Because I don't go to the movies often, I'm not negatively impacted by my emotional eating. However, this could be an issue if I associated popcorn with my routine evening Netflix binge. In that case, I'd want to identify the couch as my trigger to eat and address the snack habit head on by avoiding the TV, drinking tea, or quitting eating in front of screens cold turkey.

Common Situational Triggers:

- Stepping on the scale

- Studying

- Working

- Looking at old photos

- Scrolling through social media

- Watching TV

- Times of day, such as 5 o'clock

Danielle snacked between Zoom calls while working from home. Her job felt mundane, and nothing challenged her anymore. The empty time between meetings or scheduled events left her feeling restless, so she mindlessly reached for chocolate-covered pretzels for entertainment.

The emotion was apathy, and Danielle's trigger was downtime between work calls.

Recalling that Sarah identified frustration, guilt, and depression as her primary reasons for emotionally eating, I asked Sarah which people, places, or situations triggered her feelings. Without skipping a beat, she brought up fights with her boyfriend, Ryan.

"Our zodiac signs are both Taurus, symbolized by the bull, so we butt heads a lot," Sara stated, as if this were common knowledge. "My therapist pointed out that instead of communicating how I feel, I get defensive and snippy. But Ryan always has to have the last word, so our arguments typically end in me throwing in the towel and storming out of the room."

"Then what?" I asked, admittedly a bit too over invested in the drama.

"I replay the fight in my head, obsess over every detail, and beat myself up for not being able to share what's really bothering me. In the time between when we fight and make up, I eat so I can numb out and forget the drama for a while."

She paused to let out an exhale. "Lately, my escape has been going to Kellie's Ice Cream. I don't even care for ice cream that much, but it's five minutes from my house, and I can eat it alone in my car."

"How do you feel afterwards?"

"Annoyed with myself," Sarah grunted. "And still mad at Ryan."

"Does that frustration trigger more eating?"

"Yes. Sometimes I skip meals to make up for the calories I ate. Which, of course, leads to more poor choices."

"The longer you go without giving your body energy from carbohydrates, or *glucose*, the lower your blood sugar drops," I said, handing her the blood sugar notes from The Fundamentals of Balanced Nutrition. "When your blood sugar drops too low, you'll feel irritable and tired. You may experience what some call being *hangry:* hungry and angry."

"Definitely. I turn into a monster until I get my sugar fix."

To help Sarah identify a cyclical pattern, I sketched a table. In column one, I wrote her emotional eating trigger. The second column listed the emotion. The third, her reaction to the emotion.

Trigger	Emotion	Reaction
Arguing with romantic partner	Frustration, Depression	Eat ice cream
Eating ice cream	Guilt	Skip meals
Skipping meals	'Hangry'	Poor eating choices

Table 2.3.2

"Is being hangry a legit emotion?" Sarah asked, raising an eyebrow at my chart.

"If it's not, it should be. Anyway, now that you can clearly see your emotional eating triggers, you can either eliminate them or change your reaction," I explained. "That's what will help you develop a healthy relationship with food and reach your goals."

Your Turn

Use the feelings you experience from Table 2.31. to help you identify your emotional eating triggers. The first two rows are filled in for you as examples.

Trigger	Emotion	Reaction
Doom scrolling on social media	Depression	Comfort with sweets
Stepping on the scale	Defeat	Crash dieting

Separating Weight Loss Goals from Emotional Eating

When an Emotional Eater continues to fixate on dieting for weight loss without addressing the root cause of her unwanted eating habits, she'll continue to spin her wheels. To make progress, she must put her aesthetic goals to the side and focus on fueling properly. Over time, she can adjust how she reacts to emotional eating triggers. If possible, this may also mean intentionally avoiding the people, places, or things that lead to emotional eating episodes.

Once an Emotional Eater overcomes her emotional eating, she can determine if anything else in her diet or exercise routine can be adjusted. While this may or may not result in immediate physical changes, addressing the reasons why she emotionally eats will keep her from self-sabotaging with junk food and excess snacking. This is a crucial step for sustainable weight changes.

A Healthy Relationship with Food

"Improving your relationship to food starts with improving your relationship with yourself," I told Sarah. "This means having compassion for your struggles throughout the history of emotional eating, dieting, and your body image."

"I don't think I have had a healthy relationship with food since the third grade," Sarah groaned. "Does that mean I'm damaged goods?"

"Nope."

Sarah squinted at me, clearly skeptical of my confidence and optimism.

"I've seen people on social media talk about having a healthy relationship with food," she said. "Is that a legitimate pursuit or just a trend?"

"Both," I laughed. "The reason it's so popular right now is because many women are realizing the restrictive diets from the past have screwed with their perceptions of food."

I pulled out another worksheet titled *Signs of a Healthy Relationship with Food*. The list included:

- Listening and respecting your natural hunger cues

- Eating when you're hungry and stopping you're when full

- Giving yourself permission to eat any and all foods—nothing is off-limits!

- Trusting yourself around food

- Not relying on food to self-soothe

- The focus of food choices is not just calorie or macronutrient content

- Not needing to justify food selections

- Understanding your worth is not defined by how or what you eat

- Practicing mindful eating

- Choosing foods based on how they make you feel

"These descriptions remind me of my best friend and former roommate Kylie," Sarah said as she skimmed the criteria. "When we lived together, I noticed she kept bags of pretzels and Girl Scout Cookies in her pantry for weeks without finishing them. I never understood how she could take a few bites, put it back, and forget about it. If there's anything bad in my kitchen, I'll obsess over it until it's gone."

Sarah went on to explain how Kylie rarely overeats, only skips breakfast when she is hungover or sick, and never makes negative comments about her eating choices. When it comes to portion control, Kylie doesn't count macros or worry about what people think of her appetite. Sometimes she finishes an entire plate of food while other times she eats a third and throws it out.

"Since your mother was unable to demonstrate what a healthy relationship with food looks like, Kylie can be your new role model," I suggested. "What are three behaviors around food Kylie has that you can emulate?"

"She doesn't skip meals to save calories, she doesn't use food to cope with her feelings, and she listens to her natural hunger cues."

"How *does* she deal when life flat out sucks?"

Sarah rolled her eyes. "She jogs."

Your Turn

To better understand your relationship to food, answer the following prompts:

- How would you describe your relationship to food?

- Are there any people in your life who have a healthy relationship to food?

- What behaviors or mindsets do they have around eating that you'd like to emulate? If no one comes to mind, use the list of *Signs of a Healthy Relationship with Food* to help you.

Hyperpalatable Foods

If we only reached for celery sticks when we wanted to emotionally eat, it wouldn't be so bad, right? Maybe. But there is a reason why choosing vegetables in the heat of the moment rarely happens.

Facing our uncomfortable emotions can be painful, which is why so many people search for something outside themselves to temporarily boost their mood. One way to feel better instantly is to eat a food that is *hyperpalatable*. A hyperpalatable food is one where the synergy between the components of the food—such as fat, salt, sugar, and carbohydrates—makes it tastier than it would be otherwise.

Think of it like this: a plain baked potato tastes all right, but you probably wouldn't eat more than just one. If you thinly slice, fry, and add salt to that same potato, you've got a bag of kettle chips! Eating a whole spud with your footlong sandwich is easy when it's in chip form, yet most of us would feel overwhelmed eating an entire potato with a 12-inch sub. This is because the addition of salt and oil make the potato easier to consume in excess. Chips are less satiating but taste way better than a plain ol' tater.

Hyperpalatable foods also tend to have a pleasurable mouthfeel, such as smooth vanilla ice cream with cookie dough chunks and salted pretzels. These flavor and texture combinations hit the brain with a surge of dopamine, a feel-good chemical that does a wonderful job of helping us through tough times. This is why no one craves ground turkey or broccoli when they're emotionally eating. The dopamine response is not as strong and therefore, doesn't distract from our pain.

I notice many clients who emotionally eat when they're sad or lonely go for softer, comfort foods like cheesy pasta, soft serve, and gooey baked goods, while clients who eat due to stress or anxiety gravitate towards chips, salty trail mix, and crackers.

Think about it. The act of chewing releases built up tension. There is something therapeutic about clenching down on something crunchy, whereas the softer textures of comfort foods feel like a warm hug when you're blue.

Healthy Reactions to Emotions & Emotional Eating Triggers

No one escapes this life without stress, sadness, or loneliness. Therefore, finding proactive ways to manage heavy feelings is crucial to putting an end to habitual emotional eating.

"Other than food, what do you do on a regular basis to help you manage life's stresses?" I asked Sarah.

"I dunno," she shrugged. "Binge watch *Game of Thrones* or shop consignment."

"Coping mechanisms like TV, social media, online shopping, and alcohol are similar to food in that they distract you for a moment, but you usually walk away feeling tired or drained. They may also trigger even more emotional or boredom eating," I explained. "The best coping tools will energize you or give you a sense of release and wellbeing."

"Don't tell me I need to run like Kylie," Sarah groaned.

"Unless that's your jam, you don't have to hit the track," I reassured her. "The best coping mechanisms are the ones you *want* to do and don't take a lot of effort for you to initiate. If you *loathe* exercising, for instance, the idea of doing air squats or taking a walk when all you want to do is curl up with a bowl of noodles may seem impossible to start."

"*Just get up and take a waaaalk,*" Sarah mocked in a whiney voice. "I hate that advice. In the thick of my emotional meltdowns, the last thing I want to do is risk running into my chatty neighbors."

Even though taking a walk was my preferred self-preservation tactic, I understood what Sarah meant. I feel the same when an influencer suggests soaking a bubble bath when stressed. How is wasting time in a tub of water going to solve my problem?!

"Exercise works for some people but like most wellness tips, it's not universal," I replied. "We'll find a few strategies that work for you."

"Deal," Sarah gave me a single nod.

"When it comes to managing emotions, it's important to have *proactive* coping mechanisms and *instant* coping mechanisms," I continued. "Proactive coping mechanisms are practices you can integrate to help regulate negative emotions before they come up. This includes a morning kickboxing class to help burn off steam before you're triggered, a cold plunge[18] to build mental resilience, or meditating each morning to start each day with a sense of peace."

"Traditional therapy is proactive, too," Sarah thought aloud. "Working with a professional has given me the tools and confidence to face tough emotions when they arise, but as much as I'd love to text my therapist every time something happens, that's not reality."

"Exactly! Some tools should be *instant* coping mechanisms, which are behaviors you can turn to the moment you feel triggered. Taking deep breaths, walking out the door to stand in the sunshine, or texting a friend to vent are instant coping mechanisms. Essentially, these are accessible tools *you* don't feel resistant to starting."

I thought of my friend Nico used to use a vaporizer pen when he felt stressed because it was a quick and instant relief. When we finally convinced him to kick the habit because of the horrific health consequences, he developed a dependency on caffeine. Soon, he was drinking at least four cups of coffee per day, giving him acid reflux and insomnia. Realizing he went from one unhealthy instant coping mechanism to another, he replaced sipping caffeine with unflavored seltzer water. His lungs and stomach acid thanked him for it!

"Kylie is one of those super humans who uses jogging both as a proactive and instant coping mechanism," reflected Sarah. "She also had an anonymous Reddit account where she'd complain to strangers online whenever something crappy happened. Instead of opening the pantry, I guess I could vent into the void, too? But even under an alias, I'm not sure I want to air my dirty laundry to the entire web."

"I don't blame you. Let's brainstorm other healthy coping mechanisms to use instantly or proactively."

"Let me guess—you have a list for that, too," Sarah teased.

"Correct," I laughed, shaking off any twinge of embarrassment I felt. "List-making may just be *my* preferred coping mechanism."

---

[18] *A cold plunge is exactly what it sounds like- submerging one's body into a tank, bath, or pool filled with ice cold water. Not only can a cold plunge improve recovery after a strenuous workout, but biohackers claim the "flight-or-flight" response induced by immersing oneself in cold water helps train the brain and body to respond to day-to-day stress.*

Healthy Coping Mechanisms:

Breathwork: Breathwork is conscious, controlled breathing done especially for relaxation, meditation, or therapeutic purposes. You can search for guided breathwork practices and techniques on YouTube or use an app like Pause Breathwork or Othership. Start with 5-10 minutes of breathwork most days. If guided breathwork is too much, start with taking five deep breaths before eating.

Meditation: There is no wrong or right way to meditate! I like to start by sitting or lying with my eyes closed, sometimes in silence and sometimes to calming music. I focus on repeating one mantra such as *I am safe* or *Life is good*. Whenever my mind starts to drift, I simply come back to the mantra until I feel satisfied. This may take five minutes or thirty. Once I finish, cravings to eat or self-sabotage evaporate! If you're new to meditation, you can search for guided meditations on YouTube or Spotify, or use an app like Calm or Headspace.

Talk (or Write) it Out: If you're comfortable discussing your issue, ask a friend if you can call or text her to vent. If you'd rather keep it private, write a letter, journal, or record yourself talking through your feelings. No one ever has to read or see what you say. Confession: I tell my miniature Australian Shepard Grits all my secrets (and he never spills!)

If you're having an interpersonal issue, confront the problem with that person or persons in a healthy and safe manner. For tips, I recommend reading the book *Nonviolent Communication* by Marshall Rosenberg, PhD.

Get into Nature: As long as you feel safe, get outside every day. Plan weekend hikes, work in an outside cafe, or sit barefoot under a tree. Breathing in fresh air is incredibly healing and is an antidote for stress. The American Psychological Association notes exposure to nature can help boost mood, attention, and feelings of empathy.

Yoga: Dropping into your body and breathing through gentle yoga can help you escape the thoughts in your head driving you to emotionally eat. Bessel van der Kolk, MD and author of *The Body Keeps the Score,* encourages individuals affected by stress and trauma to practice yoga to release tension and relax. When you slow your breathing and hold poses, you can gently increase your heart rate variability to decrease stress. Yoga also helps you to open up and feel somatic sensations, which can unlock past traumas stored in the body.

Just ten minutes of yoga a day can help you feel centered before or when you're triggered to emotionally eat. If you don't have a studio near you, there are many at-home yoga instructors such as the Peloton app or "Yoga with Adrienne" on YouTube to get you started.

Physical Activity: Moving your body is incredibly effective for releasing stored tension. Dancing, walking, and stretching are excellent options when you don't feel motivated to do traditional or intense exercises like jogging, lifting, swimming, or cycling. Of course, regular exercise can help regulate your emotions.

Get Creative: Everyone should have a creative outlet to express themselves, and I will die on that hill. Before you say, *"But Kait, I'm not artistic,"* remind yourself creativity stretches beyond the realms of art class! Creativity is simply *creating for the sake of creating*. You don't need to showcase your work or try to sell it on Etsy to benefit from a creative hobby.

Writing this book and water coloring for fun are my current creative outlets. Other ideas include making artistic videos for social media pages, baking healthy treats, nail art, writing poetry, journaling, doodling, practicing make-up and hair looks, photography, digital photo art, and crafting.

Consider investing in a class or online course to refine a tactical and creative skill. For inspiration, read or listen to *Creative Calling: Establish a Daily Practice, Infuse Your World with Meaning, and Succeed in Work + Life* by Chase Jarvis.

Pause: When you feel the urge to emotionally eat, set a timer for 5-10 minutes. During that time frame, allow yourself to feel whatever comes up without using food. Cry, scream in a pillow, pray, or take deep breaths. After the timer goes off, give yourself permission to eat if you still want to, but you likely won't feel as inclined to soothe with food.

Challenge Yourself: Nothing beats the feeling of accomplishing something hard! Set a goal, big or small, and relish in the high you get when you complete it. Ideas include training for a race, talking to one new person a day, beating a personal record at the gym or at work, giving up caffeine for a week, or joining a sports team.

Volunteer: Pouring energy into other people, pets, or a cause you care about is incredibly therapeutic and regulating. Not only does helping others feel *good*, it's a meaningful distraction and it can remind you to be appreciative of everything you have.

Gratitude: When life doesn't go your way, write down three things you feel grateful for. They can be big or small: your matcha latte, the sweet neighborhood cat you feed every morning, your healthy baby cousin. Dropping into a place of gratitude allows you to assign new meaning to your problems and reflect on everything *good* in your life, giving you space between the trigger and your desire to eat. This can be done instantly or proactively!

Talk to an Expert: Invest in a professional therapist or mental health counselor to help resolve ongoing, unresolved issues that trigger you to emotionally eat.

I recommend relying on at least two regular proactive coping mechanisms (such as daily walks and practicing guitar) and two instant coping mechanisms (such as journaling and pausing).

Your Turn

In place of eating, list at least two proactive coping mechanisms you'd like to try:

1.

2.

List at least two potential instant coping mechanisms:

1.

2.

Make sure these are coping mechanisms you'd actually enjoy or have little resistance starting. I recommend journaling about these experiences in your Food, Mood, and Body Journal.

Unhealthy Coping Mechanisms

I once had a client named Rita who opened her TikTok account when she had the urge to eat out of boredom. Since the algorithm kept showing her indulgent recipes for fudge brownies or cheesy pastas, she'd close the app and make a beeline to the pantry. Not only did social media temporarily mask emotional eating triggers, it inherently became one! For these reasons Rita decided TikTok had become an *unhealthy coping mechanism* and it needed to go.

Too often, people like Nico and Rita replace one unwanted habit for another. Instead of dessert, they'll drink two glasses of wine. Rather than chips, they'll eat rice cakes. In place of waking up to play on their phone, they'll switch on the news. It's easier to respond to our desire for instant gratification with *more* instant gratification! To put an end to unhealthy coping mechanisms, we need to slow down and address the emotional eating triggers head on.

In Rita's case, her emotional eating trigger was downtime at work. She replaced her unhealthy coping mechanisms with healthy ones. Rather than snacking or opening TikTok, she began to fill this time by cleaning her home, working on her digital art business, and meditating.

Other examples of unhealthy coping mechanisms include consuming excessive amounts of alcohol, vaping, gambling, video games, online shopping, streaming shows, and even over-exercising. That being said, it's up to each individual to determine whether or not she is abusing a coping mechanism. One person may feel at peace unwinding with a glass of wine every night while another may feel it's doing more harm than good. I personally enjoy zoning out in front of trash TV once or twice a week but more than that, I feel unsettled.

A clear sign you are abusing a coping mechanism is to ask yourself how you feel afterwards. If online shopping gives you a temporary high but is followed by anxiety or regret, it's time to find a new coping mechanism.

Your Turn

If you currently practice any healthy proactive coping mechanisms, list them here.

If you don't, refer to the list above and pick at least two alternatives you'd be willing to try to help you manage emotional eating triggers.

Now list any healthy instant coping mechanisms you currently practice. If you can't think of any, refer to the list above and pick at least two alternatives you'd be willing to try to help you curb the urge to emotional eat.

Moody or Just Hungry?

"I have so much to tell you," Sarah announced without even saying hello as she marched into the office two weeks after our previous consultation.

"I'm all ears," I cracked open a lemon seltzer water, handed it to her, and closed the office door.

"First, I have a confession." Sarah took a sip of her bubbly water. "The night of our first session, I racked up a hefty bill with UberEats."

"Those delivery fees will get ya." I raised my eyebrows but quickly returned to a neutral expression. The last thing I wanted was for Sarah to feel judged or guilty. "We all slip sometimes. I have to ask, how did it happen?"

"After our session, I threw myself a pity party. It felt unfair that I have to struggle with weight and emotional eating," she confessed. "I didn't want to do all this stupid inner work to heal my relationship with food. I wanted it to be as easy as *eat less, move more*."

If it were that simple, no one would struggle with weight, I thought.

"Of course, these negative thoughts triggered me to feel frustrated and hopeless. Instead of turning to my coping mechanisms, I said, *Screw this, I'm ordering loaded nachos, cinnamon twists, and a soda,*" Sarah continued. "When I woke up, I felt bloated and defeated. It was the final straw for me. I was ready to commit to our plan."

"How'd that go?' I asked.

"The first day was the worst because I wanted to skip meals to make up for my feast, but I ignored the impulse and ate once I felt hungry. For breakfast, I had full-fat cottage cheese and sliced mangos per the BNT Protocol. Then I did a yoga flow on my back porch and wrote in my gratitude journal. Afterwards, I felt a million times lighter. Any guilt I had about the night before dissipated."

Sarah went on to tell me how she ate white bean chili for lunch and carrots with cheese and hummus as a snack. Normally, she'd be craving junk around 4 p.m. but found it easy to reach for something nutritious.

"And the weirdest thing happened, Kait. My boyfriend noticed I was in an unusually good mood for a Tuesday," Sarah said. "Other than eating balanced meals and snacks, nothing out of the ordinary happened. Normally, I would vent to him about how annoying my job is or complain about how loud he chews. It must have been because I was relaxed rather than hangry."

For Sarah, skipping meals triggered feelings of irritability, causing her to soothe with hyperpalatable food. Exhaustion and frustration from lack of food are common catalysts for Emotional Eaters.

"I have another big win," she went on. "Last Thursday, our company told us they were about to lay off ten percent of my department. Even though I didn't think my position was at risk, I felt anxious all day long but made sure I did my yoga. In an attempt to make me feel better, Ryan brought home a box of frosted cookies."

"Ooph, that's hard to resist."

"You're telling me. Ryan shows his love for me with treats and gifts, so it was hard to be upset. But here's the kicker, I only had *one* cookie! Normally, I'd devour the whole box."

Sarah explained how she had eaten three balanced meals that day, which likely stabilized her blood sugar. Because she was fueled, her body wasn't craving sugar like it normally was. Even though the other cookies looked yummy, she set a timer for ten minutes before grabbing another. By the time the buzzer went off, she had already forgotten about the cookies. The box sat on her counter for three days before Ryan threw the stale leftovers away. According to her, tossing treats was unheard of in their home.

Her wins from the past two weeks didn't end with the cookies. After getting off the phone with an aggressive client, Sarah didn't feel the same urge to decompress with chips.

"Normally, I'd hang up and make a beeline to the pantry. I'd stand there and snack on whatever I could get my paws on. This time, I stepped outside to text my coworkers about the situation. Simply venting to colleagues was cathartic, and I was able to return to work without taking a snack break. Other times, I took deep breaths and did mini-meditations. Worked like a charm!"

It's not that Sarah completely stopped experiencing cravings when she was stressed. Rather she was aware of her triggers and was able to self-soothe in others ways. Fueling with balanced meals also helped lessen the intensity and frequency of her cravings.

"Based on your recap, it seems like you're making strides towards how you ultimately want to feel around food," I replied.

She nodded. "I wasn't perfect, don't get me wrong. There were a couple of instances where I said screw it and ate chocolate. But it felt...different."

"How so?" I asked.

Sarah paused. "Well, eating the chocolate was a conscious choice rather than an emotional blackout. I was able to stop after a few pieces instead of going back for more. I didn't feel guilty afterwards, and I didn't want to diet the next day."

Throughout our six months working together, Sarah continued to make progress mentally and physically. Her emotional eating habits resurfaced when her brother got into a ski accident, but she was able to redirect her fear by remembering her coping mechanisms. She joined a yoga studio and made daily gratitude a habitual practice. She stopped skipping meals and focused on fueling her body so she was strong in her yoga practice. Over time, the frequency and intensity of her emotional eating habits declined as her relationship to food improved.

"For years, I thought being moody was just part of who I was, but it turns out I was just hungry and didn't have any outlets for my aggression other than food," Sarah laughed. "I still get annoyed at work and Ryan drives me nuts, but I know eating junk won't solve anything."

Sarah's mindfulness and commitment proved she was more in control of her emotional eating habits than she originally thought.

"You seem... lighter," I observed at our last face-to-face session. Although Sarah had always cracked jokes, they were sarcastic and skeptical in nature. Now, her energy was more playful. I noticed her shoulders were less tense (perhaps from all of that yoga!) and she no longer hid her midsection with her arms or oversized outerwear.

"I *feel* lighter," Sarah exclaimed. "Both mentally and physically. I've gotten into a routine with eating, which makes me feel less anxious around food because I'm confident I'll make better choices as long as I fuel myself. Eating this way doesn't feel like a diet, but my body is changing. My pants are too big, and that's not even the best part. As my relationship with food has improved, so has every other relationship in my life."

"How so?"

"The more patient and compassionate I am with myself, the more bandwidth I have for other people and their needs. I have more empathy at work and with my family, especially my mom."

"Oh?" I cocked my head, recalling the stories she told about her mom's negative self-talk about her body as a child.

"Through therapy, I uncovered I held a lot of resentment for my mom. I was angry at her for negatively influencing my relationship with food and blamed her for why I hated my body. It was not fair I had to bear her burdens as a kid and even though I loved her, I hated her for what she put me through. As I began to heal my own relationship with food, I realized she didn't have the tools I have. She didn't have a registered dietitian or mental health professional to talk through her feelings with, nor did she have the self-awareness to recognize and cope with her emotional eating triggers. My own journey has helped me forgive my mom and even find gratitude for her."

Gratitude? I felt goosebumps.

"If I had never struggled with food, who knows what other substance I would have gotten my hands on to work through my feelings about my dad!" Sarah continued, reading the curious expression on my face. "It could have been a lot worse, even deadly. If I hadn't had any problems to fix, would I have experimented with life-enriching coping mechanisms like exercise and self-reflection? Who can say, but I do know this journey has inspired me to become a yoga instructor. I want to teach other people how to love and live in their bodies. If I had been born with the perfect relationship to food and my body, I wouldn't have discovered this passion."

Your Turn

Once you've integrated healthy coping mechanisms for emotional eating triggers for at least one week, journal about your experience. Here are some prompts to get you started:

- How has your relationship to food changed?

- How has your relationship with your body or your self-esteem changed?

- How has your life changed? Are you inspired to try new things, experiment with new hobbies, or strengthen relationships?

Revisit these journal prompts every 1-4 weeks for 6 months.

Shadow Self Integration:

- Allow yourself to *feel* your feelings instead of suppressing them.

- Cope with your emotions in fulfilling, creative ways. Could you channel the pain of a heartbreak into a viral blog post or therapeutic painting routine?

- Take advantage of your passionate nature by throwing yourself into a healthy coping mechanism such as new skill or hobby.

- Explore the parts of you that make you feel guilty or ashamed and work with a professional to heal them.

- Embrace the fact you're a human with a full spectrum of emotions!

- Vulnerability breeds connection. Turn to trusted friends or family for support when you're struggling and notice if your relationship improves.

Chapter Takeaways

- It's normal to self-soothe with food from time to time but when it interferes with your quality of life, mental wellbeing, or physical health, it's time to address the root issue.

- Emotional eaters must work on their relationship with food if they want to kick the habit. This may mean putting weight loss goals on hold.

- Your relationship with food is highly influenced by your environment, your caregivers, your peers, and media consumption.

- Hyperpalatable foods (sugar with fat) provide instant feelings of pleasure, making them an effective yet potentially destructive tool for coping with unpleasant emotions.

- Get clear on which emotions and emotional eating triggers feed your unwanted eating habits. Common triggers can be interpersonal, environmental, or situational.

- Balance your meals to control blood sugar levels. Skipping meals and restriction can lead to low blood sugars, heightening feelings of irritability.

- Commit to at least four healthy coping mechanisms that don't involve food. Make sure two can be done proactively and two can be done instantly.

- In your Food, Mood, and Body Journal, track how often you emotionally eat and use new coping mechanisms to determine if you're making progress.

- Notice if you're using any other unhealthy coping mechanisms to deal with the same emotional eating triggers and replace these with healthy ones.

Chapter 4

The Yo-Yo Dieter

Shadow Tendencies:

- Researches different diets frequently

- Tempted to buy into quick result schemes even though she knows better

- Is either "on" or "off" a diet

- Sees food as "good" or "bad"

- Unsure how to regulate hunger or fullness

- Feels anxious eating outside of her plan

- Eats foods she doesn't like (because a diet told her to)

- Doesn't trust herself around food when she's not on a diet

Learning to Love Food

"Knock, knock," came a deep Southern drawl from outside my office.

I unlocked my eyes from my laptop to see a round, mousy woman tightly gripping a knitted tote bag hanging from her shoulder.

"C'mon in," I grinned. "You must be Maggie?"

"Yes ma'am." Maggie looked down as she stepped in, looking unsure of where to go or what to do. As I pulled out her chair, I noticed her hairline was sweating and her face was flushed a faint rosy red.

"I love your accent," I told her, attempting to ease her nerves. "Where are you from?"

"Oh, thank you," she chuckled. "I'm from a small town in Georgia. I recently moved to Florida with my husband for his job, but I used to come to Orlando as a child every summer with my Grammie."

Maggie wore no make-up to cover her light freckles and sported a flowy, sleeveless navy dress with buckled sandals. Though her style was simple, I noticed throughout our sessions Maggie had an affinity for festive earrings. On this day, she had on a pair of studs shaped like pastel Easter eggs in honor of the upcoming holiday.

As we continued getting to know each other, I was surprised by how much personal information Maggie shared with me. Maggie's mother was constantly in and out of jail for illicit drug charges, and her father was never in the picture. She'd been raised by her strict grandparents after her mother had lost custody when Maggie was only six years old.

"My Grammie ran a tight ship, and she was very paranoid about me getting into trouble," Maggie told me. "To keep me on the straight and narrow, Grammie signed me up for all sorts of after school activities. I was part of the church choir, the 4H club, and in the summer, I played softball." She paused to take a breath. "Sorry, I feel like I'm word-vomiting. If I am talking too much, just holler at me to stop."

"You're doing great," I encouraged. "Did Grammie control what you ate as well?"

"Oh, did she ever. I think that's why I'm in my 30's and still can't figure out my issues with food."

When Maggie was eleven years old, she hit puberty. Alarmed by her rate of maturation, the town pediatrician told her grandma that Maggie was above the curve for weight in her age group. Afraid Maggie would be bullied by the kids at school, Grammie wasted no time signing her up for Weight Watchers so she could "fix" the problem before starting 6th grade.

In hindsight, there was no problem. Maggie was simply developing earlier than her peers and experiencing the normal weight changes that accompany womanhood. An eleven-year-old didn't need to diet; she needed time to grow into her new body, focus on eating enough healthy foods, and live an active lifestyle. But by being thrown into the real world before she could even make her own lunch, Maggie learned living in a bigger body was *wrong* and dieting was *right*. That false belief planted itself into her impressionable psyche and haunted her throughout decades of diets.

"I'm over yo-yo dieting," Maggie huffed. "I'm over losing and regaining the same fifteen pounds. Just tell me exactly what and how to eat to lose weight, and I'll do whatever you say."

Unfortunately, spoon feeding her a meal plan would be giving Maggie exactly what she didn't want: a diet.

Your Turn

Answer the following questions:

1. Did you start dieting as a child or adolescent?

2. Do you stick to a diet for a short period of time, just to revert back into old eating habits as soon as you mess up?

3. Do you lose and regain the same weight over and over again?

4. Do you feel unsure on how to eat without following a set of diet rules?

5. Do you distrust your own judgment or intuitive cues about food?

6. Do you get anxious eating a meal that's "off plan"?

7. Do you eat foods you don't like because you think you're supposed to?

8. Do you avoid foods because a diet told you to?

9. Do you spend a lot of time researching different diets?

10. Have you asked people you admire about their eating habits, then tried to copy what they do?

11. Do you feel overwhelmed by all the diet advice out there?

12. Do you click on sensationalized headlines, videos, or posts about food or weight loss?

13. Do you compare your diet to *What I Eat in a Day* vlogs on social media?

If you answered "yes" to three or more of these questions, you may identify with the shadow tendencies of The Yo-Yo Dieter sub-archetype. This chapter will help you learn to eat without following restrictive diet rules.

Dieting is NOT for Children

"What did you learn about nutrition and healthy eating from weight loss groups?" I asked Maggie.

"Other than how to count points, I learned to skip breakfast on weigh-in days," Maggie chuckled with a hint of sadness. "If I lost weight, Grammie would be happy. If the scale stayed the same or went up, I felt like I let her down."

"Would she scold you if you didn't lose weight?" I asked.

"No," Maggie's voice trailed off. "But I could read the disappointment all over her face. When I lost weight, she was warm and encouraging. When I didn't, she gave me the silent treatment during the meeting."

Yikes, I thought. Maggie was conditioned to believe love and acceptance from Grammie had to be earned, which triggered disordered eating patterns such as skipping meals. Even as a full-grown adult, she was desperate to lose weight to please society.

"Before Weight Watchers, no one ever stopped me from eating what I wanted," Maggie continued. "Grammie kept Oreos around and never cared if I had three or four. She'd happily bring me a glass of whole milk to dunk 'em in! But after we started the program, she hid the Oreos because they were too many points."

My heart sank. Another example of a parental figure trying to do what she thought was best for her granddaughter while unknowingly teaching her to fear food.

"The only treat I was allowed on special occasions were those tasteless Devil's Food Cookies because they were fat-free," Maggie sighed. "Everything in the house from crackers to peanut butter had to be low fat for it to fit within my points."

I grimaced. The low-fat craze of the 90's was an absolute disaster. By extracting the delicious tasting fat from naturally occuring foods like peanut butter, food companies added sugar into their products so they didn't taste like garbage. Because fat has more calories per gram than sugar, this strategy fooled Americans into thinking it was the healthier choice. In reality, it left people feeling hungry and more inclined to overeat refined carbs.

"I know, it was depressing," Maggie said, reading the disgust on my face. "I didn't like them, but wasting perfectly good food was practically sinful in my house, so I ate them anyway."

"Do you still feel guilty for wasting food?" I asked.

Maggie nodded. She was a part of **The Clean Plate Club**, a nickname for those who eat past the point of fullness because they were expected to finish their plate as kids. Whether they weren't allowed to leave the table unless they ate their veggies or didn't get dessert unless every crumb was consumed, Clean Plate Club members are subconsciously wired to eat past the point of comfort. In Maggie's case, she was shamed into eating what was served because there were "starving children in Africa."

If you're a parent, I recommend reading Ellyn Satter's *Division of Responsibility in Feeding* as a guide to how to help your children become competent eaters. In her work, Satter explains both the children and caretakers' roles in meal time throughout each stage of development. Notably, children are to have full say in how much and whether to eat at all. Allowing children to listen to their intuitive eating skills lessens the risk they will overeat as adults.

Your Turn

Answer the following questions:

1. Do you feel compelled to finish all of the food on your plate, even if your stomach feels full?

2. Is it hard to save enough food for leftovers, especially when eating out?

3. Are you surprised when your dining partners are able to leave food on their plate when you can't?

4. Do you find yourself eating food you don't like or want because you don't want to waste it?

5. Do you feel guilty throwing away food you don't like or want?

If you answered "yes" to any of these questions, you may be part of The Clean Plate Club.

"I'm definitely part of The Clean Plate Club," Maggie laughed. "It physically pains me to throw food away! I rarely take home leftovers, and I never try new foods because I'm afraid of wasting them."

"Membership to the Clean Plate Club does not have to be for life," I said. "With practice, you can rewire your brain to stop eating when you're full. There are two mindfulness methods you can try."

The first method is by using the Hunger Scale in **The Perfectionist Chapter**. This involves eating slowly, without distractions, and taking the last bite when you feel between 6 and 7 on the Hunger Scale. As a reminder:

6- Somewhat Full: Stomach feels full but not completely satisfied. Thoughts of food become less intense or frequent.

7- Satisfied: Stomach feels comfortably full, and you're ready to move on to your next task.

It's helpful to set a timer with the goal of stretching one meal per day to at least 20 minutes. You heard me—the second method is to eat for 20 minutes! Having a timer will help you rest between bites so you can check in with your physical cues and stop when you've had enough.

The third method is committing to leave at least one bite of food on your plate each time you eat. While it may feel uncomfortable at first, this will teach you it's OK to walk away from food. You can combine this method with the first and second one.

If you normally eat an entire bread bowl of broccoli cheddar soup within eleven minutes, practice methods #1 and #2 by leaving a big ol' chunk of the bread bowl on your plate once you feel somewhat full. Wait 20 minutes before deciding to eat anything else. If you commit to method 3, purposefully leave one bite behind. Notice if it feels empowering to throw the food you don't want or need away. If so, relish in it!

If leaving food behind feels uncomfortable, that's OK, too! It's a new habit and way of thinking about food, so it will take some getting used to. Journal about what you're feeling, and see what comes up. With consistent practice, you'll be filling out your exit paperwork from The Clean Plate Club in no time!

Your Turn

If you are a part of the Clean Plate Club, experiment with one or all three of the following mindful eating practices for at least two weeks and journal about your experiences.

Method #1: Use the Hunger Scale to help you stop eating when you're physically full. Take your last bite when you feel between a 6 and 7.

Method #2: Set a timer with the goal to make a meal stretch for 20 minutes, pausing frequently to check in with your physical sensations.

Method #3: Purposefully leave at least one bite of food on every plate, every time.

I Love Food too Much

"What kinds of foods do you order, Maggie?" I asked, referring to her previous point about refusing to try and potentially waste new foods.

Maggie took a deep breath, then let out a long exhale. "I hate to admit it to you, but I told myself I'd be honest. My go-to's are chicken tenders, Italian subs, and Caesar salads with extra croutons. Despite all my diets, I love tasty food too much."

"Do you not believe healthy food can taste good, too?"

Maggie shrugged. "I don't even know what healthy food means. I know obvious things like broccoli and spinach are good for ya', but that's about it. Every diet seems to have conflicting advice on any food that isn't a green vegetable."

From mainstream diets like The South Beach Diet to extreme fads such as "The Grapefruit Diet,"[19] Maggie listed dozens of different eating plans she'd experimented with throughout the years. Everything she knew about health was based on diet plans, not on actual nutrition science or an awareness of her own body and food preferences.

"Before I start giving you recommendations on healthy foods to try, I have to ask if you have food allergies or intolerances?"

Maggie shook her head no.

"Medical conditions? Hormone imbalances?"

Tiny tears pooled in the corners of her eyes. "For the past twelve months, my husband and I have been trying to start a family, with no luck," Sarah sniffled. "When we went to the fertility specialist, he told me my weight may make it difficult for me to conceive. He ran some blood tests, took an ultrasound, and recommended I lose a few pounds before we try in vitro next year."

---

[19] Dating back to the 1930's, The Grapefruit Diet was based off the premise that, when eaten before other foods, grapefruits had an enzyme that would burn off fat. The diet lasts 10-12 days and includes food restrictions such as avoiding celery, white onion, and carbohydrate rich foods.

"How did you feel when you got that news?" I asked earnestly. I could only imagine how much pressure to lose weight she must be feeling. No wonder she wanted to jump head first into a crash diet.

"I panicked and immediately took to the internet to see what I should do. Of course, hours of reading about what to eat to increase my chance of conception left me feeling more defeated than ever. I shut my laptop and asked my husband to bring me chicken nuggets and fries."

Maggie blinked away the water in eyes, sat up straighter, and took a long, deep breath through her nose. "When the fertility specialist got my testing results back, he diagnosed me with Polycystic Ovary Syndrome (PCOS). His words were a mixture of relief to have explanation why I've struggled to lose weight and conceive, but also a sense of hopelessness and loss. I felt betrayed by my body, and overwhelmed by the uncertainty of navigating a hormone imbalance. Researching PCOS has only left me feeling confused and alone, but I refuse to let a stinkin' medical condition define me or keep me from my dream of motherhood. I'm here because I'm hopeful you can help me."

Polycystic Ovary Syndrome (PCOS)

Polycystic Ovary Syndrome (PCOS) is a hormonal disorder that occurs in women of childbearing age and is a common cause of infertility. The condition is marked by the absence of or irregular menstrual cycles, cysts on the ovaries, and excess male hormones known as androgens. Only your doctor can diagnose PCOS.

Depending on the symptoms or severity of a woman's PCOS, losing weight can be difficult. Women with PCOS are more at risk for having elevated blood insulin levels. Insulin is a hormone released from your pancreas into your blood. When you ingest glucose (energy), insulin acts as the key that opens cells in your tissues and allows the glucose to enter. Too much insulin in the blood makes cells **insulin resistant**, meaning cells are less efficient at accepting glucose. As a result, excess glucose in the blood with nowhere to go is more likely to be stored as body fat.

Insulin resistance is associated with Type II Diabetes and can be confirmed with a blood test from your doctor upon request. It's important to note insulin is not the same as your fasting blood glucose or hemoglobin A1C, tests used to diagnose diabetes.

A common misconception about PCOS is that women should restrict all carbs and/or fast for more than 14 hours a day. These extreme approaches often backfire and lead to overeating junk food. Women with PCOS benefit from the BNT protocol, limiting *added sugar*, and replacing refined carbohydrates with complex ones.

For women with elevated insulin levels and/or a diagnosis of type II diabetes, I provide individualized recommendations for how many total grams of carbohydrates to eat per meal and snacks. Generally, this range falls within 30-60 grams of complex carbohydrate per meal and 15-30 grams per snack. 80% of their total carbohydrate intake should contain no added sugar and provide at least 3 grams of fiber per serving. Regular exercise is recommended most days of the week. Walks count!

Supplementing with 4 grams of 40:1 myo-inositol & D-chiro inositol each day is shown to help regulate ovulatory cycles in women with PCOS, which is helpful for women trying to conceive.

Take Online Diet Advice with a Grain of Salt

Since her diagnosis, Maggie had spent hours researching weight loss with PCOS but reported feeling overwhelmed by the conflicting diet recommendations from various hormone "experts" online. When she showed me her sources, none of the accounts appeared to be experts at all! They lacked legitimate medical credentials, formal education in health sciences, and background experience working with the public in regulated settings.

"Maggie," I groaned, scrolling through her list. "You're taking your fertility and nutrition advice from influencers with no formal medical or nutrition training. No wonder you're confused and not having any luck."

I explained that while many medical and nutrition professionals use online platforms to share information, there are just as many (if not more) illegitimate "health coaches" using social media to make money selling online courses, meal plans, or group coaching.

Many brands also reach out to these online coaches to promote their products. Influencers who share discount codes for supplements and skinny teas are usually *affiliate marketers*. Being an affiliate means that for every product sold using a personalized code, the influencer gets a percentage of the sale. This motivates them to post videos recommending the product, even if they'd never use it in their personal life.

In the past years, there has been a rise in influencers affiliated with greens powders. They all do the same thing—record themselves mixing it in an aesthetic drinking glass, lie about how it tastes *ah-mazing*, and swear it's the only cure for bloat. If the influencer is attractive or convincing, people won't stop to question the validity of their claims. Desperate to look and feel better, they'll fork over $60 for a so-called quick fix before integrating sustainable diet and lifestyle changes.

After a week of choking down glorified lawn clippings, they'll realize their supergreens supplement isn't so super after all.

"My suggestion is to not take diet advice from someone unless they are a Registered Dietitian Nutritionist," I told Maggie. "We are professionally obligated to follow a code of ethics, which includes not promoting any nutrition supplement for profit without providing evidence supporting its use. Unless we want to risk losing our license to practice, dietitians will only share valid nutrition advice and won't scam you to make a quick buck."

Sketchy Supplements

Vitamins and supplements such as protein powder and fat loss pills are not regulated by The Food and Drug Administration Association. This means a company can mow the grass, turn it into a powder, put it in a pretty container, and sell it to you as a health supplement. Look for vitamin and sports supplement brands that are third-party tested. Third-party certification is when an outside organization such as NSF Certified for Sport® evaluates a dietary supplement and vouches for its quality.

"Keep in mind media headlines will often make outlandish claims about certain foods or diets to get traffic to their page," I warned Maggie. I proceeded to list examples I've seen.

Burn Fat by Going Gluten-Free

Khloe Kardashian Lost 10 Pounds with Skinny Tea

Charcoal Cleanse for Fat Detox

"You're telling me skinny teas are a waste of money," Maggie said sarcastically. "Who woulda thought?"

"*Definitely* not a scam," I laughed, matching her tone. "If that were a blog link you clicked, your website traffic would put money in the copywriter's pocket. That's why the headlines are so sensationalized."

I went on, "Inflating a health claim is one thing, but fear mongering is a whole other beast. Ever notice how some TikTok posts and YouTube ads will begin with terrifying statements to get you hooked? *Carbohydrates Cause Brain Cancer? 5 Fruits You Must NEVER Eat! Is Toxic Poop in Your Gut Making You Fat?*"

"Yes!" Maggie laughed. "The crazier the claim, the more I feel compelled to listen."

"Exactly. And as you do, the video ad will babble off more misleading information and try to sell you on their 'magic' solution," I said. "Even popular Netflix documentaries make false claims and create unnecessary commotion around foods to push an agenda. *The Game Changers* documentary convinced many of viewers that consuming meat will shave years off your lifespan while proponents of the Carnivore Diet claim eating nothing but meat is the secret to longevity."

"I've tried both of those diets," Maggie said sheepishly. "When I tried to be vegan, I felt guilty for eating eggs from my in-laws' chicken coop. Then the carnivore diet made me question if homegrown tomatoes and zucchini were why I was gaining weight. In hindsight, it seems silly, but at the time, I felt confused."

"With one party saying a plant-based diet is ruining your health and another swearing animal products are the root of all evil, it doesn't leave much to eat, does it?"

"Right," Maggie responded. "And if every seemingly healthy food is so bad, I don't know what to choose. I might as well eat a pizza with extra pepperoni and cheese-stuffed crust…"

All of the conflicting diet information infected Maggie with a classic case of *analysis paralysis*.

Analysis Paralysis

Analysis paralysis is defined as an individual or group's inability to make a decision or take action in a specific time frame due to overthinking a problem. It's often triggered by having too much data and/or obsessing over the pros and cons of each potential course of action.

A classic example of analysis paralysis is shopping for milk at a health food store. Years ago, the only options were skim, 2%, or whole cow's milk. Then soy milk came on the scene, giving consumers two choices: dairy or dairy-free. Simpler times!

These days, the milk aisle is jam-packed with different options: unsweetened vanilla almond milk, cashew milk, hemp seed milk, coconut milk, flaxseed milk, ultra-filtered milk…the list goes on. With so many brands telling health-conscious consumers their milk is supreme, it's difficult to make a quick decision *and* feel good about it.

The same is true for diets. With so many programs claiming their approach to eating is the cure-all, no wonder Yo-Yo dieters are feeling confused and overwhelmed! Proponents of Keto are telling them to put butter in their coffee while an ex-body-builder recommends low-fat spray butter on everything. Then a self-proclaimed holistic "nutritionist" demonizes both options by demanding dieters simply purchase a farm, milk their own cows, and churn butter in their free time to avoid chemicals. *Sigh*.

After listening to so many different rules, Yo-Yo Dieters like Maggie develop a superpower that is anything but super. Present them with any meal, food or recipe, and they will tell you why it's bad.

Take a quinoa salad with chickpeas and carrots tossed in an olive oil vinaigrette for example. Objectively, this meal has many health benefits. There's plant-based protein from the quinoa and chickpeas, fiber and phytonutrients from the veggies, and healthy fats in the olive oil. But a Yo-Yo dieter ignores the big picture because she's too busy fretting over every single ingredient. She thinks, *Both quinoa and chickpeas? Too many carbs. Olive oil? Too high in calories. Carrots? Too much sugar.*

By finding fault, the Yo-Yo Dieter self-sabotages. *If nothing is good for me*, she thinks, *why even try?* She's back to eating sugary cereal for dinner.

Dieting: Self-Sabotage?

By holding herself to impossible diet standards, Maggie gave herself an excuse to give up because deep down she was expecting to fail. This cycle allowed Maggie to continue self-sabotaging with food (which was a lot more comfortable than creating new habits).

In order to reach her goals, Maggie needed to mourn the part of her that ordered chicken tenders every night while embracing the new version of her who ate balanced, nutritious meals.

When I shared this insight with Maggie, she agreed.

"That happened to me at the supermarket," Maggie said. "I was shopping for the protein bars you suggested, but when I looked at the ingredients on the box, I started thinkin' all of the reasons they were bad. Even though they were made from nuts and dates, I talked myself into thinking they had too many carbs. I put 'em back just to grab a bag of chocolate peanut butter cups."

Instead of considering the benefits of protein bars, Maggie came up with reasons to put them back on the shelf. This allowed her to talk herself out of choosing the better option and rationalize buying what she actually wanted: dessert.

The secret to ending the cycle of self-sabotage is to **stop dieting.** Instead, integrate BNT Protocol to focus on the many benefits of a food, not what makes it evil. Practicing a **Benefits Mindset** encourages eating nutritious, filling food instead of fueling a restrictive mindset around eating.

Table 2.4.1 compares a restrictive mindset to a mindset that focuses on the benefits of a food.

Food	Restrictive Mindset	Benefits Mindset
Peanut Butter	Too high in calories and fat	Makes a meal or snack more satiating Curbs cravings for sugar later in the day
Hamburger Patty	Too high in saturated fat	Adds protein and iron to a meal Simple to meal prep Easy to balance with complex carbs and vegetables Loved by the whole family!
Acai Bowl	Too much sugar from fruit	Full of fiber and flavor Easy to balance with healthy fats and protein rich toppings like nuts, seeds, and coconut

Table 2.4.1

Your Turn

Identify at least two benefits of nutritious foods that are commonly restricted in popular diets. Use the last two rows to explore other foods you have restricted in the past. Examples of answers are provided at the end of this chapter!

Food	Restrictive Mindset	Benefits Mindset
Cheese Stick	Dairy is scary	
Rice	White foods are bad	
Pineapple	Fruit has too much sugar	
Bread	Carbs make you fat	

Table 2.4.2

Cleaning Out the Closet

To make room for a benefits mindset, Yo-Yo Dieters must take time to throw out all the junk they've learned from restrictive eating over the years. I call this *cleaning out the closet*.

"Following a diet begins innocently enough," I told Maggie. "You begin to pick up tips on how to eat, then store that information on a metaphorical shelf in your brain. As you continue to dabble in new diets, your collection of rules takes up so much space in your brain that your mental shelf can't hold them all. You're forced to upgrade to a storage bin.

"As the storage bin fills, you realize you need an entire closet to store all of your diet rules. The more you diet, the more information that gets stored in your closet until it begins to overflow. Soon you can't even close the door without shoving your hold body up against it. Like an episode of *Hoarders*, your brain is cluttered with so much conflicting information there is no room to accomplish anything. So you sit there in your pile, wondering what to do next."

"That's exactly how it feels inside my head," she answered, laughing. "I need a maid!"

"If only it were that easy. You can't outsource this mess with a maid. You're going to have to get your hands dirty and clean out that space yourself."

Maggie laughed nervously. "Good Lord. What are you gonna make me do?"

I stood up from my chair, walked to the other side of the office, and opened up a filing cabinet with client handouts, menus, and nutrition resources.

"We're going to do a bit of diet rule purging," I said as I thumbed through the labeled folders. "Like this filing cabinet, we're going to sort and organize your beliefs about what and how to eat. We'll only keep the approaches that are valuable and forget the rest."

I pulled out the sheet I was looking for and handed it to Maggie.

Food Rules

Years of dieting can make it hard to know which eating habits are actually helpful and which ones keep you stuck. Use this sheet to clarify which dieting rules need to go and which eating practices to keep (if any!)

1. Brainstorm a list of all the food and diet rules you have followed or are currently following.

2. Which of these rules have kept you stuck in unhealthy eating patterns and left you feeling deprived, confused, or overwhelmed? These are the rules we'll throw out!

3. Review your list. Did any of these rules help you? How so?

"The purpose of The Food Rules exercise is to help you become aware of conflicting diet rules, explore which eating habits are helpful and which ones are not, and declutter your brain from all the nonsense," I explained.

As an example, I showed Maggie a copy of a recovering Yo-Yo Dieter named Cora's answers:

1. Brainstorm a list of all the food & diet rules you have followed or are currently following.

    ○ Eating six small meals per day
    ○ Choosing only non-fat dairy products
    ○ Avoiding fruit

2. Which of these rules have kept you stuck in unhealthy eating patterns and left you feeling deprived, confused, or over-whelmed? These are the rules we'll throw out!

    ○ I never feel full after eating low-fat yogurts and cottage cheese. I just keep snacking until I'm too full for dinner!
    ○ Avoiding fruit feels limiting and counterintuitive to what I know feels good for my body.

3. Review your list. Did any of these rules help you? How so?

    ○ Eating six meals a day helped me feel less guilty about snacking. I found fueling throughout the day helped me manage my cravings for sweets and treats. However, pausing my routine to eat every 2-3 hours is not practical for me. I found eating four or five times worked best for my schedule and appetite.

The One Silver Lining of Dieting

Not every outcome of dieting is evil! From the example above, Cora demonstrates how experimenting with new eating patterns can teach us about how food impacts our bodies. By fueling six times a day instead of three, Cora discovered snacking is her friend, not foe! But when she realized eating *that* often was not realistic, she didn't blame herself. Instead, she was able to reflect and modify the rule to fit her own needs.

My client Lexi had a similar experience after attempting to eat a whopping 1 gram of protein per pound of body weight per day. Because she was filling up on so much protein, she struggled to eat enough fiber from complex carbs. As a result, she went from pooping once a day to once every two or three days. As you can imagine, she felt extremely uncomfortable!

"I don't know what to do," Lexi told me. "I heard eating all of that protein is good for me, but how can it be healthy if it makes my digestion worse?"

I suggested her intuition and body were wiser than an arbitrary diet rule she found online, and she could still reap the benefits of a high protein diet without compromising her comfort. Once she decided to moderately decrease her protein to make room for complex carbs, Lexi discovered fiber had the same impact on her satiety *and* kept her on a regular bathroom schedule.

Assessment is a Yo-Yo Dieter's competitive edge. When she can objectively look at a diet rule and decide how it affects her, she can better refine her unique approach to healthy living.

"When you're filling this sheet out, don't hold back," I told Maggie as we wrapped up our session. "No one but you and I will ever read this. It's for you to clean out the junk and create space for a healthy relationship with food."

Your Turn

Fill out your own copy of the Food Rules Worksheet:

1. Brainstorm a list of all the food & diet rules you have followed or are currently following.

2. Which of these rules have kept you stuck in unhealthy eating patterns and left you feeling deprived, confused, or overwhelmed? These are the rules we'll throw out

3. Review your list. Did any of these rules help you? How so?

Too This, Too That

I walked into the lobby of my office building soaking wet from a Florida summer rain. Despite moving from Missouri to Orlando four years prior, I still hadn't adjusted to the afternoon showers and often forgot to bring my umbrella. Luckily, I had a hooded sweatshirt in my car and was able to protect my blowout from getting totally ruined. I stomped my feet on the welcome mat and began to slip the damp hoodie from my head when a voice around the corner startled me.

"I ran out of space, so I wrote in the margins."

Maggie was sitting in the lobby, fifteen minutes early for our scheduled session. She had swapped her Easter egg studs for beaded 4th of July firework earrings. At first, I had no idea what she meant until I saw her unfold and smooth out her Food Rules worksheet.

"Wonderful," I sighed, one hand on my pounding chest as my heart rate returned to normal. "Sounds like you did some deep mental cleansing. Let's head into my office."

It had been three weeks since our first session, but we went back and forth via email. Although she was extremely motivated to change, she continued to feel overwhelmed by diet culture.

In one of our messages, Maggie wrote:

> *I'm sending you this email panickin'. I had a Caesar salad for lunch, which has 40 grams of fat! I'm in my head about what a portion is. Is it alright to eat that much fat with dinner?*
>
> *Sincerely,*
> *Maggie*

The email communicated a lot more to me than just what Maggie had for lunch. I could tell she was allowing previous diet rules to make her feel guilty. I was afraid she'd think, *Screw it, I already messed up* and make a poor decision at dinner.

I replied:

Maggie,

> *No need to panic. Sure, Caesar salad dressing isn't the most heart healthy source of fat, but you don't need to restrict yourself from eating a balanced meal at dinner to make up for it. Using the BNT protocol and your Food Rules Worksheet, consider the following questions:*
>
> 1. *What diet rule around fat is coming up for you?*
>
> 2. *Is it a helpful rule or a harmful rule?*
>
> *-Kait Richardson, RDN, LD*

Within minutes, she answered:

> *On my last diet, I was only allowed a total of 30 grams of fat per day. It made me fear eating dietary fat with meals. I've learned from the BNT Protocol that eating*

foods with fat earlier in the day keeps me out of the cookie jar!

To round out the day, I'm going to try to make an ahi tuna poke bowl with brown rice and tons of pickled veggies. I normally use spicy mayo but this time, I'll swap it for a heart healthy fat such as avocado. For a kick, I'll down that bad boy in hot sauce!

By slowing down and eating more balanced and nutritious meals, Maggie was focused on the big picture. Making healthy adjustments later would continue to fuel her body. This shift needed to become habitual if she was going to stop mentally collapsing every time she second guessed whether what she was eating was *too this or too that*.

To practice balancing meals, I asked Maggie to send me a list of her favorite comfort foods. Then, I sent her ideas on how to make them more nutritious.

How to Balance Comfort Meals

Modify...	By...
Caesar salads	• Replacing romaine lettuce with a leafy green like dinosaur kale • Adding grilled chicken • Using a dressing made from a Greek yogurt base
Fried chicken tenders	• Using an air fryer
French fries	• Baking sweet potato fries for more fiber and Vitamin C • Tossing in a heart healthy fat such as avocado oil
Egg noodles with butter	• Using a pasta made from chickpeas, lentils, or black beans for more fiber and protein • Adding grilled shrimp for additional protein
Mango sorbet	• Preparing a mango and chia seed pudding made with unsweetened coconut milk
Brownies	• Nothing! Dessert alternatives suck. Simply enjoy a brownie following a balanced meal

Table 2.4.3

Pasta from chickpeas? Maggie wrote back. *If you say so…*

Your Turn

Using The BNT Protocol and lists from the Fundamentals of Balanced Nutrition chapter , modify the following comfort meals to boost the satiety and nutrition content.

Modify...	By...
Mac n' Cheese	
Veggie Sushi Roll	
Strawberry Banana Smoothie	
Italian Sub Sandwich	

Table 2.4.4

Suggestions for modifications are listed at the end of the chapter.

Once I was settled and able to review Maggie's Food Rules Worksheet, I realized she was not joking when she said she ran out of space.

Maggie's list of rules included:

- *Whole30: No sugar, dairy, legumes, alcohol, or grains*
- *Processed foods are off limits*
- *No red meat*
- *No more than two eggs per week*
- *No white carbs such as pasta, bread, or white rice*
- *Limit fat to less than 30 grams per day*
- *Avoid all fruit except berries*
- *Don't eat anything from a package*
- *No eating in front of a screen*
- *Chew each bite 30 times before swallowing*

Sheesh! No wonder she was scared of eating; everything was off limits. Plus, some of these rules made eating a chore. Sure, it's nice to eat at a table without distractions but when there's a tight deadline, dining at your desk may be the only option. And chewing each bite thirty times? Ain't nobody got time for that!

I also noticed Maggie had restrictions regarding when to eat:

- *Don't eat three hours before bed*
- *Intermittent fast for 16 hours per day*
- *Eat breakfast within one hour of waking up*

If she were to follow all of these rules at the same time, she'd be eating her first meal around 7 AM and stopping at 3 PM. Even for the old folks at the nursing home, a 3 p.m. dinner time is too early and impractical!

"I found myself feeling bad for waking up hungry," Maggie admitted. "But guilty if I ate or didn't fast in the morning."

The guilt was her first clue these rules were not working. The other was that they simply *were not working*.

The second section of the worksheet asked her to explore which rules made her feel deprived and why. While nearly all of her answers from the first section were listed, one reflection caught my attention.

Avoiding all processed foods has kept me from making nutritious meals.

"I feel like every gosh darn food is processed," exclaimed Maggie when I asked her to elaborate. "Even guacamole and canned beans are technically processed. Even though I know deep down they are nutritious, labeling all processed foods as bad kept me from making simple yet balanced meals."

Processed Versus Ultra-Processed Foods

Labeling all processed foods as "bad" is misleading. Instead, think of processed foods and ultra-processed foods. While both processed and ultra-processed foods have undergone modifications, you must consider the differences in ingredients, processing level, and nutrition between the two.

Ingredients in processed foods may contain sugar, fat, or salt for flavor enhancement or shelf-preservation, but they still contain ingredients that are recognizable such as a can of black beans with added salt and seasoning. Ultra-processed foods have ingredients you wouldn't find in a home kitchen such as artifical flavors, colors, sweeteners, and hydrogenated oils.

The **processing level** in processed foods having been adjusted by means of cooking, packaging, freezing, drying, or canning. Baby carrots are technically processed from whole carrots to make them more aesthetic and palatable to consumers. You won't find baby carrots in nature but unlike ultra-processed foods like frosted cereals or sports drinks, they contain no additives, preservatives, artifical flavors, fake sweeteners, or funky chemicals.

Depending on the added ingredients and processing level, the **nutritional value** remains high in many processed foods. In other words, the vitamins, minerals, fiber, protein, antioxidants, or phytonutrients remain high in these foods. Examples include frozen fruits and vegetables, salted nuts, energy bars made from dates and nuts, cheese sticks, and protein powders with no added junk. Ultra-processed foods tend to be low in essential nutrients yet high in saturated fat, refined sugars, additives, or sodium. Examples include sugary granola bars, pre-packaged snacks and desserts, fast food, or boxed Mac n' cheese.

Swapping her restrictive mindset with a benefits mindset would allow Maggie to replace ultra-processed foods like candy with nutritious alternatives like fruit and nut bars, even if they were minimally processed.

Like Cora, I wanted Maggie to reflect on any benefits from past diets. To do so, we referred to the third section on her Food Rules worksheet where she was asked to reflect on which eating practices from past diets served her in some way. Maggie liked:

- *Not eating three hours before bed*

- *Whole30*

"I learned lying down for bed after eating doesn't bode well for my heartburn," Maggie explained. "So that rule helps me limit late night snacking."

Before I could ask about Whole30, she read my mind. "Trust me, I know Whole30's rules are out of control. I mean, no legumes? I love beans! But following that diet helped me in two ways."

"Ok, spill the beans!" I couldn't resist, the set up was perfect!

"For one, it forced me to cook instead of relying on take-out. I got real familiar with the kitchen, which impressed my husband. Whole30 also helped me discover I don't need a beer every day after work to unwind. I would have never thought I could go an entire month without a cold one," she chuckled.

"Cheers to that!" I winked.

Fuller Than a Tick

Maggie was forced to postpone our third appointment to stay with her half-sister June in the hospital after she suffered a massive heart attack.

"I'm sorry to hear that," I said sympathetically when she told me the news over the phone. "I didn't realize you had a sister. Are you close?"

"Not really," Maggie replied. "She's thirteen years older than me, and she lived with her papa while we were growin' up. But neither of us have any surviving family left, so I'm about all she's got."

"I'm glad you are able to be there with her."

"Lord knows I am too," she sighed. "I will say, being in the hospital only motivates me to stick to my healthy eating goals. Heart issues run in my family, and I don't want my future baby to have to watch me suffer like this."

"I know it's hard to be mindful when you don't have access to your own kitchen. How are you managing?"

"Surprisingly well," Maggie replied. "We're staying at my sister's house at night, so I'm able to fix a healthy supper and breakfast before we head for the hospital. The lunch options at the cafeteria aren't all that great, but I can make do with the salad bar if I bring my own can of tuna to mix in. I'm also not afraid to grab a minimally-processed protein bar if I need a snack. Normally, I'd use this stressful trip as a reason to eat at the local diners, but I am committed to staying on track. We did have Chick-Fil-A once, but I ordered the grilled chicken wrap with fruit instead of my usual crispy chicken sandwich, fries, and BBQ sauce. I only ate about two thirds before I threw it away. I was fuller than a tick!"

I was proud. Maggie wasn't allowing old fears about processed foods to prevent her from relying on healthy foods like canned tuna or protein bars, nor did she use her unforeseen circumstance as a reason to slip back into old eating behaviors. Instead of creating rules around what not to eat, she was finding ways to incorporate the foods she needed to change.

Though we had a follow-up scheduled one week after our chat, Maggie informed me she decided to extend their trip and work remotely from Georgia for a while. It turns out her sister was a bit of a hoarder, and Maggie and her husband wanted to help clean out her home.

"It's the right thing to do," Maggie told me when she called to reschedule. "Plus, a cluttered home makes a person feel stressed. That ain't good for her heart. If it's alright with you, I'll schedule an appointment when I'm home and settled."

I told her that it was fine as long as she cleaned that home like she did her closet of diet rules.

Jumpin' Bean

For unexpected reasons, our third meeting would be our last for the year. It had been months since we chatted in-depth, but nearly every update Maggie sent to me was positive.

"Hi Kait," Maggie said as she bounced into my office in a sunflower yellow dress. This time, she sported a pair of bright orange pom pom earrings. While she was usually in a good mood, she seemed particularly chipper this morning.

She plopped down in the chair, sat on her hands, and rocked excitedly back and forth. Although she had always dressed in vibrant colors, something about her look felt brighter. Maybe she had a tan? Or a new shade of blush?

"Look at you!" I admired. "You're glowing. What are they serving up in Georgia?"

"Must be all of 'em fruits and vegetables I've been eating," she laughed as she playfully patted her stomach.

"What else has improved since we started meeting?" I asked, anxious to hear what else was making Maggie skip into my office with a happy grin slapped on her face.

"Gosh! Where do I even begin," she started, her smile stretching wider. "Since we first met four months ago, I've felt more confident about grocery shopping and ordering food. That feels great! I also invested in new cookware since whipping up healthy meals has gone from being a chore to a hobby. You'll also be happy to know I am enjoying chickpea pasta, too."

"I never thought I'd see the day!"

Maggie chuckled and then, as casually as reminding me of a rescheduled lunch meeting or a new episode of Love is Blind, she shared she was pregnant.

I let out a gasp and almost leapt out of my chair. "You're what!?"

Maggie pressed her lips into a smile and nodded.

"*That* explains why you're glowing!" I exclaimed.

"I know, I can't believe it," Maggie subtly shrieked. "My period was late which is not uncommon with PCOS, but my husband insisted I take a pregnancy test anyway. Sure enough, the little stick read positive. We were shocked, so I took three more, and they all confirmed our suspicions. I'm about eight weeks, meaning our baby is the size of a jumpin' bean!"

On day one, Maggie shared with me how her main goal for her health was to be able to conceive. Regardless of how her diet changes and initial weight loss made a difference, she had gotten pregnant. I couldn't stop telling her how excited I was for her.

"Thank you," she beamed. "It's still early, so we haven't shared the news to many people yet. But I have to tell you, old habits die hard! I've had to stop myself from obsessively reading about PCOS pregnancy stories online. I find myself getting worked up and anxious when I read what women are saying is good or bad for the baby."

I nodded in agreement. Similar to diets, there is a lot of conflicting and unsolicited advice surrounding fertility and pregnancy floating around the internet. The last thing a vulnerable woman needs is more stress from online chatter.

"I don't need to clutter another closet with information," Maggie chuckled. "Instead of worrying, I'm going to get all of my information from a few credible sources and listen to my own instincts."

"I like that perspective," I smiled. "Too much stress is never good for your body, and it especially isn't good for your baby."

For the remainder of the session, Maggie and I discussed general nutrition recommendations for a healthy pregnancy. We agreed her weight loss goals were to be put on hold, and her main priority was to provide her baby with adequate nutrition to support healthy development.

Maggie no longer needed to supplement with 4 grams of myo-inositol while she was pregnant, so I told her to replace it with a daily prenatal vitamin and 200mg DHA (docosahexaenoic acid)·

Since Maggie had new food aversions to most meats and Greek yogurt, she incorporated protein from whey protein pancakes, beans, and lentils to meet her needs. Although she didn't have morning sickness, her intermittent nausea made it hard to eat every 3-6 hours.

"I'm less strict on the timing of when I eat," Maggie admitted. "I just eat when I can stomach it. I still don't eat before lying down, though. My acid reflux is out of control!"

To help her blood circulation and improve her fitness level for childbirth, she decided to add in thirty minutes of walking three times a week and sign-up for a prenatal yoga class. There was no reason for her to start strenuous exercise during pregnancy, but restorative movement would help her feel better and build healthy habits.

"Starting this journey in spring was perfect timing," Maggie shared with me the last minutes of our last appointment. "I came in wanting to lose weight, and obviously those goals are on hold, but learning how to trust my body and quit blindly following diet rules is much more important."

I asked her to elaborate.

"Before our sessions, I had never taken the time to trust and listen to my body. Instead, I dieted. I tried to control every little thing I ate in an effort to change it, but that just left me feeling more out of tune with my needs. Throughout this journey, I've been forced to slow down, reflect on my own needs, and fuel myself with foods that feel good." She patted her belly lovingly. "Now I'm pregnant, and all I can think about is how my body feels, the subtle shifts, the nausea! If I had started this journey alone, I think I'd be less accepting of my unpredictable appetite, the cravings, and new food aversions. I would have tried to override my body's cries with rules, rules, and more stinkin' rules. What good would that do?"

"Absolutely none," I answered. "You would just be stressed and overwhelmed during a time you should be calm and at peace."

"Exactly. I've discovered self-compassion and self-reflection work best for me," Maggie said. "And when the baby does arrive, I'll have both the confidence to fuel myself without a diet and the energy to focus on the baby's needs."

Shadow Self Integration:

- Previous diet recommendations may have value. Explore which ones help you, which ones you need to let go, then actually let them go!

- Researching nutrition and eating strategies can be helpful, but make sure you're consuming content from reputable sources such as registered dietitians or peer-reviewed studies.

- Modify meals to be more nutritious instead of more restricted.

- Use your intuition and body cues to help you determine whether or not a certain diet approach is working for you or not. If the diet says eat at noon but you're not hungry, trust your body and wait until later.

Chapter Takeaways

- Yo-Yo Dieting can ultimately stall your progress because it leaves you feeling confused and overwhelmed with how or what to eat.

- Membership to The Clean Plate Club doesn't have to be for life! Practice eating slower and purposefully leaving food behind to break the habit.

- Analysis paralysis from excessive researching can make you feel confused and prevent you from taking targeted action towards your goals.

- If a diet or weight loss claim seems too good to be true, believe it.

- Just because a food has been processed doesn't mean it's unhealthy. Check the ingredients, processing level, and nutrition content.

- Setting food rules that are impossible to follow is self-sabotage.

- When it comes to food, focus on what *to* eat (benefits mindset) instead of what *not to* eat (restrictive mindset).

- Clean out your cluttered mental closet with a brain dump of all of the diet rules you've followed or currently follow. Identify which ones made you feel deprived and which ones, if any, have helped you.

Suggested Answers to 2.4.2 and 2.4.4

Table 2.4.2

Food	Restrictive Mindset	Benefits Mindset
Cheese Stick		Adds protein and calcium to a meal Makes a low-fat meal satiating
Rice		Cheap and easy to make in bulk Pairs well with fibrous veggies
Pineapple		Adds fiber and flavor to protein shakes Contains enzymes to help with digestion
Bread		Fiber-rich varieties promote satiety and healthy digestion Provides energy

Table 2.4.4

Modify...	By...
Mac n' Cheese	Stirring in roasted broccoli for additional fiber
	Replacing cheese with a butternut squash sauce for additional fiber and micronutrients
	Adding grilled chicken for protein
	Using a chickpea pasta for additional protein or fiber
Vegetarian Sushi Roll	Ordering a side of edamame for extra protein and fiber
	Increasing avocado for additional satiety
Strawberry Banana Smoothie	Including Greek yogurt or whey protein powder
	Stirring in natural nut butter for satiety
	Adding chia seeds or ground flaxseeds for Omega-3 fatty acids
	Blending with a nutritious milk such as hemp seed milk
Italian Sub Sandwich	Use whole a grain bread
	Replace mayo with healthier fats such as avocado or hummus
	Swap salami with leaner proteins such as roasted turkey or chicken
	Add tons of veggies like tomato, spinach, pickles, and onion!

Chapter 5

The Binge Eater

Shadow Tendencies:

- Often eats one way in front of others and another way in secret

- Overeats in response to uncomfortable emotions or situations (often waiting until alone to do so)

- Turns to food to satisfy emotional needs such as pleasure, comfort, or connection to self

- Feels ashamed about eating habits

- May attempt to diet or restrict food after binge eating episodes

- Compares personal eating habits to habits of others

Lighten Up!

Standing at 5'10", my client Josie had a larger than life presence. Her thick, tangled red hair and powerful build reminded me of an Amazonian version of Merida from the movie Brave. Unlike my client Mila who dressed in the most elegant of athletic clothes, Josie showed up in mismatched floral gym shorts and graphic muscle tanks. This made it impossible not to notice her cushiony, muscular quads and broad shoulders, both suggesting she knew her way around a Crossfit gym or power rack. I rarely noticed her wearing make-up to cover up her acne scars or small blemishes but if she did, it was light and undetectable. Josie unapologetically owned who she was.

Despite her warrior-like stature, Josie was a golden retriever at heart. Each appointment, she'd trot in wagging her invisible tail with the same energy as a dog eager to play. Josie's joyous outlook, infectious smile, and enthusiasm for self-improvement were contagious, even when things didn't go her way. I wanted to bottle up her happy-go-lucky spirit and unleash it on my clients who adopted a more pessimistic approach to healthy living.

Working with Josie never actually felt like work. Throughout our nine sessions, we'd chit chat as if we were two friends grabbing oat milk lattes after a pilates class. We'd joke about Mercury being in retrograde as the reason her InstaCart grocery delivery vanished and roll our eyes at wellness influencers promoting unregulated probiotic pills on TikTok. Since she was usually my last appointment on Wednesday evenings, I didn't feel pressure to end our sessions right at the end of the allotted thirty minutes.

But Josie wasn't meeting with me to make small talk. Admittedly, she had battled poor body image most of her life, and her ongoing binge eating habits weren't helping. She was sick of feeling like "the big friend" and wanted to gain control over her eating habits. She was referred to me by her therapist who wanted Josie to learn how to fuel her body to boost her self-esteem.

"I recognize being skinny won't automatically improve my confidence," Josie told me when I asked her motivation to lose weight. "One of my closest friends, who happens to be thin and drop dead gorgeous, has the self-image of a hobbit."

"I'm not familiar with the self-perceptions of fictional elves, but I'm guessing it's not good?"

"Hobbits are not elves, but good try," Josie's laugh rang so loud I was sure the tenants across the building could hear us through both the walls and sound machine hung outside my door. "My friend is a literal bikini model. At her bachelorette party in Vegas, she had a few drinks and broke down about how she thinks she is fat and ugly. My brain couldn't understand how this woman in front of me who is undeniably stunning could speak of herself that way. I tried to hype her up by reminding her we were there to celebrate her bachelorette party, and there was no reason to be upset, but she was not having it. We ended up staying in the hotel that night and watching movies."

"It's true that being thin isn't synonymous with having confidence," I told her. "But following through with healthy lifestyle goals day after day can definitely boost morale. The ticket to confidence is not the size of your jeans. It's proving to yourself that you can do hard things again and again."

Enthusiastically, Josie agreed. She explained how she's experienced high levels of self-confidence in other areas of her life, including work, mental health, and fitness. As a young adult, she struggled with depression, anxiety, and escaped two abusive relationships. Right after she left her last boyfriend, she committed herself to regular therapy and resolving her childhood traumas, including her father having a second family he seemingly cared about more than her and her sister. During her healing process, she fell in love with the squat rack and found the weight room to be extremely cathartic.

"It's the eating part I struggle with," she confessed. "Once the coronavirus pandemic hit, I used food and wine to cope. While nothing was open, I'd use going through the drive-thru as an excursion and pick up food at least once per day. At night, I'd treat myself to wine in front of the TV or video calls with friends. Even though the lockdown is over and I'm back in the gym, those unhealthy habits have stuck around."

Josie wasn't the only one whose rocky relationship with eating got worse after the pandemic. Years have gone by, and I continue to have clients making appointments with goals to shed COVID-19 weight.

"I'm not a loser, but my eating habits make me feel like one," Josie confessed. "I worked really hard to accomplish my dreams before turning thirty. I paid my own way through college, finished my Master's degree in Accounting, and I'm making bank at my company. In fact, I was told today that I am a shoe-in for an executive leader position being posted next week!"

"Make that money, girl!" I cheered and brushed my palms together as if I were throwing dollar bills in the air.

"Yeah, I'm a legit boss," Josie laughed. "On the outside, I have it all together. I have a great career, friends, and even own my own home. But when it comes to food, I feel like a mess. When I told my therapist about my eating habits, she suggested I see a dietitian to address my binge eating."

Binge Eating

Although Binge Eaters overeat, not all overeaters are Binge Eaters. Overeating every now and then is normal and doesn't disrupt one's quality of life or self-esteem. It usually happens on special occasions, when you can eat after a busy afternoon with no breaks, or when the food is just too dang good!

Binge eating, on the other hand, is compulsively eating an excessive amount of food frequently enough that it negatively impacts your sense of self or physical wellbeing. Binge eating is not associated with compensatory behaviors such as taking laxatives or purging after meals, as seen with bulimia nervosa.

Per the National Eating Disorders Association website, a binge eating episode is characterized by the following:

- Eating, in a discreet period of time such as one hour, an amount of food that is clearly larger than what most people would eat in a similar period of time under similar circumstances

- Lack of control over eating during the episode (e.g., a feeling that one cannot stop eating or control what or how much one is eating). They may feel like they're zoning out.

Binge eating episodes are also associated with three (or more) of the following:

- Eating much more rapidly than normal

- Eating until uncomfortably full

- Eating large amounts of food when not feeling physically hungry

- Eating alone because there's embarrassment by how much one is eating

- Feeling disgusted with oneself, depressed, or guilty afterward

- Marked distress regarding the binge eating

- Binge eating at least once a week for 3 months

Other warning signs of binge eating include hoarding food, rearranging one's schedule to make time for binges, obsession over weight and weight fluctuations, fear of eating in public, and frequent checking of one's self in the mirror.

If you've experienced three or more of these criteria, does that mean you have Binge Eating Disorder (BED)? Not necessarily. Binge eating and BED are different, just as having an anxiety attack does not mean one has Generalized Anxiety Disorder.

Binge Eating Disorder can only be diagnosed by a psychiatrist or medical professional. If you suspect you have a binge eating disorder or any eating disorder, visit the National Eating Disorder (NEDA) website https://www.nationaleatingdisorders.org or call or text the NEDA hotline **(800) 931-2237 for help.**

I explained to Josie that only a psychiatrist or medical doctor could diagnose her with Binge Eating Disorder (BED), but she didn't need a formal prognosis to begin improving her relationship to food and eating habits. I gave her a questionnaire to better assess her struggles and binge eating tendencies provided in the journal prompt below.

Your Turn

Here is the questionnaire Josie was provided to assess her binge eating tendencies. Circle any statement applies to you:

- At least once a week, I eat past the point of comfort (a "10" on the hunger scale)

- At least once a week, I feel out of control around what or how much I am eating

- I tend to eat large amounts of food very quickly, especially when I am alone

- I zone out when I eat large amounts of food quickly

- I want to eat even when I am not physically hungry

- I eat certain foods or amounts of food in secret because I am embarrassed by what or how I am eating

- After eating, I feel ashamed or disgusted with myself for hours or days

- I hoard food

- I fear eating in public or in front of other people

If you have experienced any of the above at least once a week for over three months, you may identify with

The Binge Eater sub-archetype. While the strategies in this chapter will help you correct any of your unwanted eating habits, I strongly recommend you reach out to a Registered Dietitian, mental health professional, or medical doctor for one-on-one support.

"Which binge eating behaviors do you exhibit?" I asked Josie.

"I definitely feel out of control around food more than once per week," she replied. "And I eat past the point of comfort, usually alone at home or in my car. While I don't hoard food, I'll go out of my way to pick something up. Afterwards, I feel embarrassed and guilty by how much I ate in just one sitting. I feel like a fraud."

"A fraud?" I questioned.

"Yep. How does a successful woman and fitness freak like me struggle with eating so damn much?"

Root Causes of Binge Eating

While every person I work with has unique experiences, there are common themes among overachievers who binge eat.

Busy women with packed schedules are left with no mental or physical energy to think about fueling well. Tracy, a single mom with a 45-minute commute from her sales job, has less time and motivation to prep, cook, and eat healthy meals than her sister Bridget who has no children and works from home. While Bridget has energy to cook salmon and veggies, the thought of making one more decision feels impossible to Tracy. Instead, she decompresses after a long day of work and child-rearing with an entire frozen pizza and a massive bowl of frosted flakes.

In this case, Tracy's binge eating comes from:

- Hunger, because she did not fuel herself throughout the day

- Seeking comfort from food

- Decision fatigue

Similar to emotional eating, the root cause(s) of binge eating can vary. Resolving them requires radical self-awareness. One Binge Eater may discover her binge eating occurs simply because she does not eat enough satiating foods during the day and resolves the problem by committing to The BNT Protocol. In this case, the root cause is related to her lifestyle.

Lifestyle causes of binge eating:

- Lack of time to eat during the day, leading to massive cravings despite knowing what's healthy & what's not

- Prioritizing emails over meals

- Not taking breaks during the day to eat or rest

- Feeling too stressed to eat, rest, or exercise

- Appetite suppression from caffeine or prescription drugs such as amphetamines, followed by overeating in the evening or on weekends

- Yo-yo dieting or restrictive eating

Setting reminders to eat, scheduling meal breaks, setting personal and professional boundaries, and holding off on coffee until after a meal can help ensure your body is fueled and limited the risk of binge eating later. If time is limited, prepping meals and snacks in advance can help. Make it a priority!

Your Turn

If you're a Binge Eater, answer the following questions.

1. Are some or all the root causes of your binge eating lifestyle related? If so, list examples.

2. What needs to change in your current routines and boundaries to prioritize fueling throughout the day?

Stress Hormones & Weight Gain

Making time to rest and recover from the day's stressors can be more effective for weight loss than cramming in a workout. Cortisol, the body's stress hormone, is secreted during intense exercise. While this is beneficial in short bursts, it can be detrimental to women who are experiencing chronic levels of stress throughout the day. This is because elevated cortisol is linked to increased belly fat, cravings, and increased appetite.

However, I find many of my most stressed clients are addicted to high intensity exercise! When I suggest taking a break from bootcamp or long-distance running, they panic because working out makes them feel less anxious. I tell these women they don't need to ditch high intensity training completely. Rather, they should replace between 25-75% of these workouts with lower impact ones.

Restorative exercises such as walking, yoga, bike riding, or pilates can simultaneously keep you fit while reducing stress. Even switching from heavy lifting to low impact weight training can help you maintain muscle without stressing the body. For even more psychophysiological benefits, take your workout into nature or with friends.

Other root causes to binge eat are emotional and psychological, sometimes requiring additional treatment from a mental health professional.

Emotional and psychological causes of binge eating:

- Seeking emotional comfort from food

- Using food as a distraction from stress or chaos

- Using food as an outlet for suppressed emotions and/or personal traumas

- Low self-esteem

- Depression

- Poor body image

- Perfectionism

As Josie and I combed through the reasons she struggled with food, it became clear most of her binge eating issues stemmed from her busy lifestyle, loneliness, and low self-esteem.

Your Turn

If you're a Binge Eater, answer the following questions:

1. Are some or all of the root causes of your binge eating emotional or psychologically related? If so, list how.

2. Which practices in your life are helping you overcome emotional eating or low self-esteem?

3. What other ideas have you considered to help you manage emotional eating or low self-esteem?

Revenge Body

"Even though I am busy, getting to the gym is not a problem for me," Josie reinforced. I could tell Josie took a lot of pride from being committed to exercise, which made me wonder if she made it a point to tell everyone about her workouts as a way to distract from her less healthy habits.

"What kind of workouts do you do?" I asked.

"I hit the gym after work five days a week. Squat, deadlift, bench press... you name it, I lift it." Josie beamed. "When I first started weight training seven years ago, I could barely squat the 20 pound metal bar but just last week I hit a new personal record of 250 pounds."

Heavy lifting five days a week for seven years? I thought. Even though I was no stranger to the gym, my joints could never!

"When I was in grad school and didn't have a budget for booze, take-out, or steak houses, I lost quite a bit of body fat with my routine," Josie reminisced. "While I don't miss eating pouch tuna and crackers every day, living off student loans was a pretty effective diet. Soon after I began to make big girl money, the pounds crept back on until I got my heart broken. I unwillingly discovered getting dumped is another shitty yet powerful way to temporarily drop weight."

She wasn't wrong. After break-ups, people showcase pictures of their "revenge bodies," claiming they've been in the gym and watching their diet to get revenge on their ex. My guess is this is to get the attention of ex-lovers and make them regret losing them!

While these so-called revenge bodies are achieved from hard work, they could be the result of having no appetite due to depression. I told Josie how my lowest adult body weight was after breaking up with my first boyfriend in college. "I had too much anxiety to eat and locked myself in my room to nap during lunch. As soon as I got over him, my appetite returned and my weight rose back to its healthy baseline."

"Same here, except it didn't stop at a healthy baseline," she said. "As soon as I felt better, I was out with friends eating and drinking every night. When I'd be home alone, I'd treat myself to whatever sounded good. Burgers, tacos, milkshakes... Admittedly, that was three years ago, and I haven't exactly stopped."

"I'm guessing your steady salary as an executive accountant makes the chance you're settling for saltines and canned fish unlikely?" I asked.

"*Almost* executive," Josie corrected me. "I don't want to jinx it! But you're right, the smell of *Chicken of the Sea* would trigger post-traumatic stress symptoms within me, so I'd rather not."

"Tell me what you eat and drink, then," I asked.

Josie's face flushed and her upbeat expression sunk ever so slightly. "I told myself I would be completely honest if I came here," she said courageously. "I know lying about my eating habits won't help."

I nodded in agreement. The last thing I want from my clients is for them to tell me what they *think* I want to hear, not what they actually eat. Trust me, I can read through the BS.

"I usually eat really clean."

"I literally crave salads."

"Yum, yum, baked chicken! I can't get enough."

Oh, please! No one likes baked chicken enough to eat it every day. And if they did, eating clean (aka, flavorless) could be why they're struggling with consistency.

"First confession that nobody knows, I love fast food," Josie admitted. "I know the meat is probably synthetic, but I could eat a quarter pounder with cheese and McDonalds fries for breakfast, lunch, and dinner."

Josie went on to tell me how she usually goes through a drive thru at least once most days of the week.

"It sounds pathetic but the thought of getting a treat motivates me to roll out of bed and start work in the morning," Josie shrugged. "I think, *If I get up right now, I'll have time to swing by a Dunkin drive thru*."

She must not have a dog. Or a baby. Nothing like a loud, dependent creature crying for your attention to stand in as the 5 a.m. alarm clock.

"And if you don't get Dunkin?" I asked.

"Then I don't eat," Josie shrugged. "I'll sip iced coffee until I have time to stop work. Sometimes it's at noon, but most days I don't eat until about 3 p.m. Either way, I'll order something healthy like a salad."

A salad, I thought. *Just because a salad has lettuce and no croutons doesn't mean the meal is balanced or nutritious.*

"Do you eat anything before you go to the gym?" I asked.

"I normally chug a pre-workout supplement or an energy drink on the way," she said.

I gently scolded her for treating caffeine as a replacement for food.

Energy Drinks are NOT Fuel

Zero-calorie energy drinks and caffeine should not be replacements for fuel from food. Unlike food, which provides calories and/or carbohydrates (glucose) our muscles can use for energy, caffeine is a stimulant. Stimulants increase brain activity, increasing the circulation of cortisol and adrenaline. This is why after drinking coffee, pre-workout powders, or energy drinks (which can contain over twice as much caffeine than a cup of coffee), many people experience a buzz and assume its energy. But without pairing caffeine with glucose, the body's cells are not receiving ready-to-use fuel to function.

Once caffeine has been metabolized, the body also experiences a crash. This causes cravings for...

- sugar and refined carbohydrates (because they are quick sources of energy)

- a nap

- more caffeine!

Some energy drinks contain nutrients such as amino acids or electrolytes, which cleverly disguises them as "health foods." Absolutely not! You're better off getting those nutrients and more from *real* food.

If you insist on drinking energy drinks every now and then, fine. Just promise me you won't use them as replacements for actual food.

Recalling how heavy Josie said she lifted, I was shocked she was disciplined enough to get into the weight room with so little gas in her tank. While her commitment was admirable, I was concerned for her joint health. Before I could ask, Josie went on to tell me she leaves the gym feeling ravenous.

"I rarely make it home without having to stop somewhere to pick up food, even if I have healthy meals prepared at home," she said, looking rather defeated. "Whenever I swear not to get fast food, I never make it through the week."

Each time Josie went on a health kick, she'd go all-in by pre-prepping her meals for the entire week. For days she'd eat baked fish and brown rice out of Tupperware, but as soon as she had a stressful day, she'd throw it out and rack up a big bill on her way home from the gym. Her personal record? Spending $37.77 at Taco Bell!

"Seven-seven-seven is my angel number," Josie stated without a hint of irony in her tone.

"Oh?" I raised my eyebrows.

"Yes! Seeing three sevens in a row is a sign from the heavens that you're living in alignment, and you're exactly where you need to be. I took it as a signal I was meant to go home and eat Nachos Bell Grande alone!"

I must have been wearing my confusion on my face because Josie interrupted my silence.

"I know it sounds silly, but it made me feel better in the moment."

"How'd you feel afterwards?"

"Anything *but* aligned," Josie chuckled. "Every time I binge, I feel puffy and bloated. I'll stand in front of the mirror and lift my shirt up to inspect the damage. I don't know why I do it, it only makes me feel worse."

What Josie was describing is known as **body checking**. Body checks are compulsive behaviors where one seeks out information about her body weight, size, and condition. While everyone looks in the mirror before a date or heading out the door to work, body checking can become problematic when repeated too frequently, especially if it causes negative self-talk and anxiety. It can also lead to disordered eating patterns such as restrictive dieting, binging, purging, and/or overexercising.

In many ways, body checking is a self-fulfilling prophecy: a woman thinks she is too fat so she inspects her tummy after eating to confirm this is true. Feeling bad, she restricts the next day just to end up binging out of shame and starvation. In Josie's case, I suspected her "inspecting the damage" was a way of affirming deep rooted beliefs about her body. If she consciously or subconsciously believes her body is flawed, body checking after an overeating episode would confirm that idea. The dark side is that body checking may intensify negative beliefs, triggering more disordered eating.

"How do you feel about your body?" I questioned.

"Could be worse," she shrugged.

"What do you mean?"

"Well, I like how I can see my muscle definition. I have powerful legs, which I get compliments on all of the time," she said, her faint smile quickly turning flat. "But for all the work I put in the gym, I feel as though it should be more obvious. I see how my fit friends eat, and they don't over or under-eat. Most of them are in relationships, too. They must not binge on fast food like me. If I quit binging, I'd look like them."

"How do you know your friends aren't regularly binging, too?" I asked.

"I don't know." She sniffed. "But given how skinny they all are, it's doubtful."

"I've had women of all shapes, sizes, backgrounds, relationship statuses, and ages come into my office and share their struggles with overeating. If there is one thing I can say for sure is that you never truly know how someone eats behind closed doors, regardless of their body size."

Josie opened her mouth to speak, then paused. After a few beats, she asked me if these women lived alone or with partners. I replied, "Both."

"But don't you think living with a significant other makes it harder to hide poor eating habits or binging?"

"Not necessarily," I replied, thinking of how Mila The Perfectionist snuck generous bowls of gelato as a midmorning snack when her husband left for work. "If some people can hide affairs or bank accounts from their spouses, others can surely hide candy wrappers."

Josie laughed, mentioning she saw plenty of shady business working in finance.

"Speaking of romantic lives," I continued. "I noticed you continue to mention how your small-bodied friends with assumingly small appetites are in relationships. Why is that?"

By the look of her face, I had caught Josie off guard. For a brief instant, I felt bad. No one expects their dietitian to ask them personal questions, but my job is to encourage people to consider not only what to eat but *why* they eat. Simply suggesting substituting chips for raw broccoli is not going to help if the person devours a sleeve of Pringles because they're lonely.

To discover the root cause of Josie's binge eating, we needed to roll up our sleeves and dig.

The Dig

"Why does it matter?" Josie deflected my question. Her tone went from sweet to sour, her body language from open to closed. She folded her arms across her chest, pointer finger tapping nervously on her sleeve, and chewed on her bottom lip. I had stepped next to a land mine, and if I didn't choose my words carefully, it would detonate.

"I'm sorry, I didn't mean it as an insult. I'm only curious if there is a connection between how you associate body weight with relationship status. We don't have to talk about it if—"

"No," she sighed. "We should talk about it."

Josie went on to explain how her entire life she had been the "big" friend in social groups. "The first time I was aware of my size was in 3rd grade. My best friend Courtney was very petite while I was ahead of the curve on growth. I'm not sure where this stemmed from, but she'd sing to me a made-up rendition of Nelly Furtado's song *I'm Like a Bird*. It went like, *I'm like a whale, I cannot fly awaaay.*

"Courtney would sing it in front of our classmates, and the boys would cackle and make up their own lyrics. I'd pretend to think it was funny, too, but it stung. I'd go home and cry."

"That's awful," I said, putting my hand to my chest. "Not even clever. Little kids are cruel."

Josie half-smiled. "Well, we talked about it a decade later. Courtney felt so bad and swore she didn't know she was hurting my feelings. She just liked making the other kids laugh. Unfortunately, the song evolved into a nickname that followed me throughout middle school. Even though I ran with the popular girls, the boys called me *Shamu*. Since no one wanted to date the girl who was bullied for being overweight, I watched as my friends got male attention while I didn't. When we'd go to the movies, I'd sit at the end while everyone else paired up with their crushes. Luckily, my friends went out of their way to include me on group outings and school dances, but I was always the single one. I also happened to be the fattest one."

My heart sank. From the sidelines, Josie witnessed her peers experience their first kisses and relationships while she longed for the same. At sleepovers, Josie pretended to be excited about the flirty notes her friends received while silently questioning why no one was blowing up her instant messenger.

The only reasons Josie could come up with were based on what she observed. What did her friends with boyfriends have in common? They were thinner. Therefore, Josie assumed if she weighed less, she'd be worthy.

Worthy of attention.

Worthy of love.

Worthy as a woman.

All based on something as fickle and cheap as the teenage male gaze.

"It didn't help I was in school in the 2000s," Josie continued. "Low-rise jeans were trendy, and the only women I saw in fashion were a size two on a bad day. You know, the Olsen twins, Lindsey Lohan, and Christina Aguilera. I distinctly remember reading a *People* magazine that quoted Mandy Moore saying she wished sample sizes in the model industry included *regular* sizes instead of only zero's and two's."

"Well, she was ahead of her time," I said.

"That's not all she said." she chuckled. "Ms. Moore's definition of *regular* was a size six or eight. As a size twelve, I was crushed. The next day, I begged my mom to buy me Slim Fast and a membership to the YMCA."

"How'd that go?"

"Actually, it worked. The summer before freshman year, I would use the elliptical for sixty minutes most days and replace two meals with a bar or shake. Within three months, I was swimming in my old clothes! My mom had to buy me a whole new wardrobe. I'll never forget how confident I felt that first day of high school."

"Did the boys notice?"

"*Everyone* noticed," Josie said, her eyes widening. "That year, I got my first boyfriend, Sam. He had gone to another middle school and didn't know me as Shamu. We dated on and off most of high school, and I still consider him my first love. He encouraged me to join the field hockey and lacrosse team, which explains why I was able to stay trim after I ditched the shakes. It was only when I discovered alcohol senior year that I quit sports and regained weight. Sam wasn't into partying, so we broke up."

"Have you been in a relationship since Sam?"

She shook her head. "I've had flings, but the men I date don't want to commit to me."

I took a moment to reflect on Josie's history. She grew up thinking her weight was why boys didn't like her. This false belief was reaffirmed once she found herself in a relationship the moment she lost weight. After she regained the weight, she found herself perpetually single again. I worried she was creating a self-fulfilling prophecy: lose weight or die alone. Our shovel was breaking ground, but we hadn't hit the root cause of her binge eating behaviors.

"How do you feel about being single?" I asked.

"I'm so freaking sick of it," Josie laughed. "Have you been on dating apps lately? They're a disaster."

Having been a user of dating apps myself, I shuddered at the memory of weird conversations and awkward first dates. "They're definitely a hit or miss. Do you feel ashamed about your relationship status?"

"Maybe?" She drew out the syllables, thinking as she responded. "Shame feels like a harsh word but maybe. You know, society expects women to be married with kids by thirty. It was always my plan, but I'm not even close. When I see my friends living the life I always pictured for myself, I feel depressed and hopeless."

"When do these feelings come up the most?"

"When I'm home alone in the evening, especially after going out with a group of friends and their partners."

"Does the feeling of loneliness make you want to eat?"

"Everything in sight."

Now we were getting somewhere.

One of the root causes of Josie's binge eating was emotional. When she felt lonely, she ate to feel better. Then, she'd wake up feeling guilty or gross. In an effort to feel better, she'd eat "clean" and workout. Of course, she'd wind up feeling hungry after a long day. Her restrictive eating was a physiological root cause of her binge eating, and only added fuel to the emotional fire.

"You know, women of all shapes and sizes are in happy relationships. Even the most beautiful, fit women find themselves feeling lonely, too. Trust me, I hear it all the time."

"Really?"

I nodded vigorously. "Oh yeah. I've had loving couples come in, and the woman lives in a larger body, but her partner dotes on her because he loves her for everything she is. I've also had supermodel clients cry to me about how their ex-boyfriends criticize their thighs. And I've heard everything in-between. My conclusion is, body size is not correlated to relationship status or quality. If your partner only loves you because of your weight, he's not the right one."

"Everyone says that," Josie said. "But I struggle to believe it. If it were true, why don't I have a boyfriend? I know I'm likable. I have tons of friends and close relationships with my family."

As is the case with many Emotional Eaters and Binge Eaters, what Josie was truly hungry for went beyond food. What she craved was deep connection, companionship, and self-love.

Your Turn

Reflect on your root causes of binge eating. What are you actually hungry for?

You, Ronald, and The Gym: A Toxic Love Triangle

"Are you saying Ronald McDonald is my stand-in boyfriend?" Josie replied when I suggested that fast food played a bigger role in her life than just dinner.

"You tell me," I stated. "I'm only throwing spaghetti on the wall to see if it sticks."

Josie pursed her lips as her gaze shifted, signaling she didn't like what I was saying but was considering the possibility.

"For a long time, I loved lifting weights," she began. "So much so, I often joked the only man I'd date is named *Jim*."

"Who is Jim, er, the gym, to you now?" I prodded.

"More of a routine, I suppose," Josie sighed, slouching in her chair. "I like lifting, but I don't get butterflies before a workout like I used to."

I knew exactly what she meant by butterflies. For years, I experienced a rush of adrenaline walking into the weight room. It was like the honeymoon phase of a relationship; every workout started with a rush of nervous excitement, and I couldn't imagine I'd commit to another type of exercise. For years I followed the same routine at the gym, forcing myself to lift even if I was sore or having period cramps. I was so afraid that changing my routine would result in a loss of progress.

But when the pandemic hit and all of the gyms shut their doors, I was forced to dabble in other types of fitness. I downloaded a guided running app and began jogging and practiced yoga on my apartment balcony. When I woke up full of energy, I'd challenge myself with a hard run. When I felt achy and stiff, I gave myself permission to do a low intensity yoga flow. For the first time in my life, I was listening to my body instead of a rigid program.

As soon as the gym reopened, I returned the gym only part time. Introducing novelty into my fitness routines allowed me to live a fuller, more satisfying life. I felt challenged, connected to my body, and fit in ways I never expected. I learned a valuable lesson: breaking out of a stale pattern is good.

Since Josie was hungry for connection and self-love, I wanted her to explore new routines and activities that would fulfill those needs.

Exercising: A Pass to Binge?

"It makes me sad to say this, but I *am* growing tired of my gym routine," Josie said after hearing about my experience. "But I'm scared that if I stop, I'll gain weight from all the fast food I eat. Lifting heavy justifies all of the calories I binge afterwards."

Josie and I locked eyes for a moment, both processing the weight of what she just said: *exercise justifies a binge.*

"I end each lift obsessing about what to eat," Josie finally said after a moment of silence. "I order a ton of food and don't stop when I'm full because in my mind, I earned it. If I skip a workout, I feel guilty about what I ate the day before."

"Dang, Sherlock Holmes. You just uncovered another root cause of your binge eating."

Your Turn

Do you exercise solely for the purpose of burning calories?

Do you also justify overeating or binge eating because you exercised?

If you answered yes to either question, reflect on how overexercising may be a root cause for binge eating.

"Other than junk food, is there anything else you look forward to after the gym?" I asked.

"Sometimes I treat myself to a few White Claws."

Josie's current routine was mundane and didn't provide her with any novelty or new outlets for connection. Sure, her mind was occupied at work and the hour she hit the gym, but with six empty hours to kill before bed, Josie had an opportunity to replace unwanted eating and drinking routines with new activities that fed her soul what she was truly craving.

"There's no denying how valuable exercise and movement is for your mental and physical health, but I want you to consider different methods you can try that are less likely to trigger a binge."

"I tried a pilates class once," Josie said. "But I felt out of place. Many of the women in my class were petite, wearing only sports bras to expose their flat, toned tummies. I felt like they were judging me by my oversized T-shirt and leggings."

"Did feeling judged trigger you to binge eat?"

"Sure did," she huffed and leaned back in her chair. "I went straight down the street for a peach milkshake and a fried chicken sandwich. Are you sure you're not a shrink?"

It's not uncommon for Binge Eaters to discover their own judgmental thoughts can lead them to binge. Afterall, who feels *good* after beating themselves up?

"Definitely not a shrink. I know the weight room is surrounded by mirrors, so it's impossible not to stare at your body while you lift. Does that make you feel insecure, too?"

"I think it does, but in a different way than pilates," Josie responded. "Even though I am not comparing myself as harshly, there are days I am hypercritical about how I look."

Nobel Prize-winning scientist Daniel Kahneman says we experience approximately 20,000 moments every single day. The quality of our life is then determined by how we recognize and categorize our moments as positive, negative, or neutral. By purposefully filling our days with moments that provoke positive self-talk, Binge Eaters can reduce the frequency of their self-induced binges.

"Hear me out," I began. "It's important you exercise, but your commitment to the gym may be doing more harm than good. Not only are you using your hard work-outs as an excuse to eat whatever you want, you're in an environment where you judge your body more than you celebrate it. Combine those with feeling hungry and lonely, you're destined for a binge. When you finish eating, negative thoughts come back with a vengeance, and the cycle continues."

Josie groaned and hung her head. "I can see how I'm self-sabotaging."

I proposed Josie begin to explore activities that could challenge her while giving her connection.

"That idea feels equal parts exciting and overwhelming," Josie admitted. "I don't even know where to start."

It was time to explore *Flow State*.

Flow State

If you're feeling overwhelmed by the idea of adding positive situations into your life, take a deep breath. Not every day needs to be packed with hobbies, meetings, chores, or extracurriculars. There is value in boredom, and making time to relax is crucial. But, if your idea of relaxing is sitting in front of a screen with a bag of SunChips, you may be experiencing unwanted consequences. (FYI- SunChips are *not* healthier than traditional potato chips. Nor are pretzels or veggie straws). In this case, it's time to push yourself to get up and *do something*.

I once had a 40-something client named Maddy who identified gardening as a positive activity in her life. She loved the feeling of digging in the dirt and the satisfaction of growing her own food, but despite months of daydreaming about tending to a home garden, Maddy claimed she had no energy. After the stress of managing a real estate brokerage and parenting ten-year-old twins, all she wanted to do after work was kick her feet up and melt into a pint of ice cream. Week after week, she felt a looming sense of disappointment that she didn't touch any of her home gardens and masked her sorrows with more dessert.

"Energy is a cycle," I preached. "If you eat like crap, you'll feel like crap. A big bowl of sugar isn't going to help you spring out of bed the next morning and tackle the day. You have to bypass the urge to sit on the couch and push yourself to go outdoors."

It's rare for anyone to step outside their comfort zone without kicking and screaming. The childlike voice in your head will be begging you to revert back to your old ways, even if you logically know that doing so will provoke more negative-self talk. The brain loves comfort, which is why pushing past the resistance can feel impossible.

To combat this feeling, it's crucial to start small when replacing an unwanted eating or lifestyle habit with a healthier one. By setting smaller, seemingly useless goals, the resistance that comes with starting and repeating a new habit shrinks.

In the past, Maddy was setting big goals around her afternoon routine. She'd tell herself she could not have any ice cream nor could she watch TV until she gardened for at least one hour. By the time she was supposed to grab her shovel, the thought of working in the sun for sixty minutes felt overwhelming. Suffocated by analysis paralysis, Maddy mentally collapsed and did nothing.

She needed to change her expectations to invoke positive self-talk instead of negative self-talk. Clearly, one hour was too much and restricting food was demotivating. To decrease Maddy's resistance to starting, she simplified her goal: before watching TV and eating ice cream, she was to spend five minutes outside in the yard.

Whether she was researching on her iPad in the grass or physically planting flowers and seeds, Maddy only had to commit to 300 measly seconds in the dirt. Then, it was up to her how she wanted to spend the rest of her evening. Her only goal was to *begin*.

Three weeks later, Maddy waltzed into my office with her chin held high.

"I only had ice cream once this month!" She gloated. "I found that changing into my gardening clothes before picking the kids up from practice encouraged me to get outside instead of making a beeline for the couch. Once I start, I don't think about stopping until my husband hollers at me to eat dinner."

Gardening put Maddy in a *flow state*[20] When someone is in flow, they are so immersed in a project, task, or creative pursuit that they lose track of time! A passionate pastry chef is in flow while she bakes, an inspired author while she writes, and a dancer while she twirls. Their minds are focused on one task and one task only, and they are not distracted by thoughts of food or negative self-talk. Afterwards, they feel accomplished, boosting their self-worth.

To reach a flow state, it helps to feel well rested and fueled. Engage in an activity at a level that challenges you but doesn't make you want to give up too soon. If the task is too easy or difficult, you will not be able to maintain flow. Also be aware that a flow state is easily

---

[20] *Flow state is a deeply fulfilling state of consciousness. Learn more about how to access this part of your brain by reading the Book* Flow: The Psychology of Optimal Experience *by Mihály Csíkiszentmihályi*

interrupted. E-mail pings, text message alerts, and background noise from the TV are distractions, and act as barriers to starting an activity.

It requires intentional effort to shut off these potential interruptions and feed your soul the activities it's hungry for. Like Maddy, you will walk away feeling nourished and less inclined to binge eat.

"Digging in the dirt feels so *human*," Maddy gushed. "I feel more connected to the Earth and myself because I am following my passion. When I do decide to watch TV, it's rewarding knowing I accomplished something ahead of time. I don't feel the need to snack as often while I relax."

By pushing herself to *start* small, Maddy was able to accomplish big things. As a result, her appreciation for herself grew while her cravings shrunk. She was living in alignment with her true self!

Other examples of activities that can ease you into a flow state include drawing, cleaning, researching a topic of interest, scrapbooking, journaling, learning an instrument, having a meaningful conversation, playing sports, or practicing a new language.

Your Turn

Which activities, projects, or tasks have you done, currently do, or would like to try to put you in a state of flow?

Just as Maddy changed into her gardening clothes and promised herself to work for five minutes, how can you decrease the resistance to starting these activities?

Leveraging Your Values

I asked Josie if she had experienced a flow state. She admitted she could not think of anything that made her feel like time didn't matter.

"Great, this is a new opportunity to discover parts of yourself that you may not know exist!"

"Your positivity is borderline toxic," Josie laughed. "But okay, hit me with your best shot. What do you suggest?"

"When we structure our days around what matters to us, we're more likely to stick to our healthy routines and feel good about it," I said. "We can best define what matters to us as our *personal values*."

"Okay…" Josie said. "I think I know where you're going with this. Someone who values kindness will feel awful if she flicks someone off in traffic, while someone who values power may feel good."

"Exactly," I said. "Our values determine how we live and how we feel about our actions. Identifying your values can give clues on how to structure time. Someone who values creativity, beauty, and service is not going to feel fulfilled sitting at home watching TV all day in her sweats. Perhaps she would if she created videos to help women with their skincare routine or designed virtual closets for friends who desperately need support elevating their personal style."

"That reminds me of my cousin Bri. She's always blabbing about 'living in alignment' or following her true calling. Apparently, her true calling is co-hosting a podcast with her best friend where they discuss reality dating shows like *Love is Blind*. To build a big audience, she invested in audio editing courses and marketing coaches. It all makes sense because she values achievement, personal growth, and quite frankly, gossip!"

I nodded in encouragement. "As much as I don't condone snarking on public figures, it's clear Bri lives by her values. Let's find yours."

I pulled up a list of personal values to show Josie, clarifying this wasn't a comprehensive list, and she could likely find examples with a simple Google search.

- Fun/Adventure

- Pleasure

- Service/ Compassion (for self and/or others)

- Family/Friends

- Love/Purpose

- Health/ Personal growth

- Achievement or Success

- Creativity

- Fitness/Movement

- Security or Safety

- Connection/Community

- Nature

- Beauty

- Freedom

- Sexuality

- Self-expression

- Money

- Animals

Based on the list, Josie identified her top values as connection, pleasure, movement, family, and animal welfare.

Your Turn

List your top ten values. Put a star beside your top five values.

Josie's next step was to think of activities to help her live in accordance with her values and reduce her reliance on food for distraction. I encouraged her to think of related activities that would challenge her while also boosting her mood and baseline level of dopamine (more on this in Chapter 6).

"Uhhh," Josie stuttered. "I'm stuck."

"Would it help if I shared examples from my own life?"

Josie nodded.

"Some of my values are creativity, friendship, movement, nature, and communication," I started. "With reflection, I realized I've held these values since I was kid! Not surprisingly, my favorite childhood hobbies were finger painting, playing in the neighborhood creek with my buddies, and going to theater camp. I've since mimicked these activities to fit within my adult life."

"You still finger paint?"

"No," I chuckled. "But I did sign up for painting classes at the local art school. Instead of playing in the creek, I explore new trails with my dog on weekends. For work, I turned my passion for performance and public speaking into The Nutrition Awareness Podcast[21]."

To help Josie come up with ideas, I forwarded her a list of life-enriching activities, projects, and tasks my other clients have adopted:

- Golf lessons

- Paddle-boarding

- Painting

- Walking and run clubs

- Online courses

- Stock trading and investing

- Coaching kids' sports teams

- Meeting other parents at playgrounds while kids play

- Writing or journaling

- Volunteering with religious or spiritual groups

- Book clubs, online or in-person

- Professional meet-ups and organizations

- Political campaigns

- City boards

- Virtual cooking lessons

- Opening Etsy shops

- Bartending certifications

---

[21] *Listen to The Nutrition Awareness Podcast on any and all podcast platforms!*

- Crafting

- Spiritual practices such as astrology, tarot card reading, or energy healing

- Virtual reality games

- Coding classes

- Vlogging and blogging about passions such as traveling, dog training, and cleaning

- Flipping houses

Family Affair

If you find yourself using parenthood or work as an excuse to avoid new things, you'll self-sabotage. Can your kids join in your hobbies? Can a family member babysit for an hour while you take time alone each week? Be creative and consider what you can make fit within your current routine.

"As excited as I am to try new things, I feel like a loser," Josie admitted. "I've spent so much time wasting away in front of dumb shows and eating chicken nuggets."

"If you're a loser for enjoying TV, that makes two of us," I reassured her. "TV is entertaining, and it can definitely fit into your life. But like junk food, too much of a good thing can cause problems. Streaming Netflix all night leaves less time in your life to explore other interests, meet new people, and create the life of your dreams."

"Good thing I only have two episodes of *Schitt's Creek* left. After the finale, I'll commit to starting a new evening routine," Josie confidently declared.

"Every single week night?" I raised an eyebrow. The last thing I wanted was for Josie to get burnt out after a week. She needed to set SMART goals.

"Eh, probably not." Josie stroked her chin. "How about for one month, I won't get fast food or turn on TV for at least three nights of the work week."

Bingo. She had found the sweet spot between challenge and ease.

"Any idea on what childhood Josie would have done in her free time?"

Josie shook her head but reassured me she would brainstorm in her manifestation journal over the weekend and report back by the following Friday.

Your Turn

List your favorite childhood activities.

Which ones align with your top five current values?

How can you mimic what you loved to do as a child in your adult life?

Can you include family or friends?

One Week Progress

Five o'clock Friday was quickly approaching, and I had yet to hear from Josie. I decided to check in before I left the office to see if she had experimented with new weekday routines. Within the hour, I got a response:

Kait,

I was just about to message you.

After our chat, I narrowed the list of values to my top five: connection, pleasure, movement, family, and animal welfare. I decided to use these values to shape how I spend my time.

Instead of going through a drive thru after my workout last night, I invited my sister and our friends over for dinner and poker. I baked us a yummy salmon filet with roasted Brussels sprouts and sweet potato gnocchi. I can't even remember the last time I had a satisfying, home cooked meal that didn't leave me wanting a bunch of junk food afterward. One of the girls brought store bought cookies, and I didn't touch them! I think it was because I was so distracted by the game, which we've decided to make a regular occurrence.

Since I love pets, I signed up to volunteer at an animal rescue every Monday and Thursday. I always wanted to, but I was too scared to skip the gym. I've noticed I'm less fixated on food on the days I am at the shelter, likely because I am not hyper focused on my body. However, I'm still active with the puppies!

Although I was a couch potato on Wednesday and Friday, I surprised myself by picking up burrito bowls for dinner instead of fast food. While I think I overate a little, I didn't binge. Still a win in my book.

This past week has given me so much hope. Thanks for sharing with me the tools I've been desperately searching for. I can't wait for our next sesh!

Xx Josie

Josie had embodied her values of connection, pleasure, and family by cooking delicious meals for her friends and sister followed by a game night. By volunteering at a local animal shelter, she remained active, even if it wasn't in the traditional sense. I was impressed.

We agreed to schedule her second session in two weeks, so she had enough time to see how her new routines impacted her binge eating.

Dog Days

"Wait until I tell you what happened the past few weeks," Josie busted into my office seven minutes early. I nearly choked on my RxBar.

"What?!" I said covering my lips with my fingertips to hide the dates in the bar that were stuck to my teeth. There's no graceful way to eat those sticky, delicious things.

Josie hung her bag on the hook, plopped down on the gray chair in front of my desk, and folded her legs criss-cross applesauce. She was sporting a matching jewel-tone sweatsuit dressed up with gold layered necklaces, hoop earrings, and stacked rings.

"To start, I've only had fast food three times since our last meeting." Josie flashed a smile and held up her phone screen displaying an impressive tally of how many days she stuck to her SMART goals. "I know that may seem like a lot for health nuts like you, but it's nothing compared to how much I was eating before."

"That's excellent!" I cheered and meant it.

"This may be TMI but after two weeks without fast food, I swooped by Chick-Fil-A while I was out running errands. Within minutes, I had to pull over at a gas station and make a run for the bathroom. It's as if my body was rejecting all of the grease."

"Sounds like your body prefers meals with more fiber and less refined oils," I said, laughing as I crumpled up my wrapper and tossed it in the trash.

"Kait, you're not kidding." Josie's face suddenly became serious. "I'm starting to actually crave healthy food. I look forward to my sprouted grain breakfast sandwiches at home and sautéed Brussels sprouts with dinner. Cooking and grocery shopping puts me in that flow state you described."

"I love it! Have any of these shifts changed how you feel about your body?"

"It may be all in my head but I just feel *lighter*," she said. "I still have bad body image days, but I don't let them linger. I am so freakin' proud that I am fueling well and living a full life, and therefore not binging, it helps me feel better about myself."

"What's your current relationship status with the gym?"

"Complicated," she laughed. "Forcing myself to go to the gym each day wasn't helping me get fit, mentally or physically. I was working out to either burn the calories from the previous night's binge or to give me permission to pig out again. While I don't plan on breaking up with the gym completely, cutting back to two or three times per week has helped me maintain the muscle I've put on without missing out on life."

"How so?" I asked.

"My fear of gaining weight guilted me into going to the gym each day instead of stepping into my community, trying new things, and connecting with people outside of work," Josie explained. "Which reminds me of the second update I wanted to share with you! Just two shifts into volunteering at the animal rescue, I have decided to adopt a dog!"

She whipped out her phone to show me photos of a stocky, 8-year-old pit bull mix with pointed ears named Bruno. Though I consider myself a professional, I am not above pausing a client session to fuss over cute dog pictures.

Even though Josie wasn't exercising in the traditional sense, walking her puppy and working in the animal shelter were keeping her active and out of the house. In these environments, she was less focused on what others thought of her body and less triggered to suppress judgmental feelings with food.

"There's more." Josie put down her phone and clasped her hands together in front of her smirk, bracing me for exciting news. "On weekend mornings, I've been walking Bruno to the dog park. It's only a half mile from my place, and we stop in a local coffee shop. Well, there's this cute guy who has been there with his pit bull at the same time. We began chatting it up about our dogs, and he asked me where I fostered Bruno."

Smiling, I could see where this was going.

"Long story short, he thought it was dope that I helped at the shelter, so I invited him to volunteer with me." Josie grinned. "We coordinated a time that worked for both of us. We're meeting for a weekend shift this Sunday morning! He suggested we meet for coffee beforehand since I always come to the park with an almond milk latte, and he wouldn't want me to short fuse because I haven't had my caffeine fix."

"Ooo, Josie has a *daaate*," I playfully teased and bopped side to side in my seat.

"Stop it," Josie grinned, her freckled cheeks blushed. "I don't want to jinx anything, but it seems like a date. No matter what happens with this guy, I feel really proud of myself for stepping outside my comfort zone."

Although I didn't say it aloud, I hoped Josie would have a positive dating experience to reinforce the idea that she was worthy of romance and love no matter if she lost weight or not. By living in accordance with her values, she had a positive energy and a newfound confidence in herself. *That* was attractive!

The Fitness Tracker Discrepancy

My clients love to show me how many calories their fitness trackers say they burned. Oftentimes, they'll link this data with health or food tracker applications to see how many calories they can eat. My response? Don't care.

Stanford Medicine found seven popular fitness trackers (Apple Watch, Basis Peak, Fitbit Surge, Microsoft Band, Mio Alpha 2, PulseOn and the Samsung Gear S2) overestimate calories burned in a workout by a whopping 27-93%!

To put this number in perspective, if your fitness watch says you burned 500 calories after a HIIT workout class, there's a likelihood you actually burned between 35 to 365 calories. That's a pretty wide gap! If the assumption that your fitness tracker is correct causes you to justify having an extra scoop of ice cream, then you may be in a caloric surplus rather than caloric maintenance or deficit.

Some of my weight lifting clients use their goal of building muscle as a reason to eat more. While it's true one must be eating enough total calories and protein to build muscle tissue, eating *too* much can also cause unwanted fat gain. Don't use a hard workout as an excuse to make poor eating decisions.

Your goal with exercise should not be to burn a specific number of calories. Pick a goal such as building muscle or improving your mile time, then train in a way that helps you reach these goals. If you don't have any specific performance goals, simply choose an activity you enjoy. If your fitness tracker or Apple Watch becomes an obsession, take a break for a month and see how you feel.

Ebb & Flow

"I am scared my newfound confidence won't last forever," Josie confessed toward the end of our session. "What if I begin to depend on fast food again or fall into old binge eating habits?"

Her worries were valid. Experiencing a taste of freedom after years of food obsession, overeating cycles, and/or dieting behaviors can feel too good to be true. But with self-awareness, Josie would learn to redirect herself when the urge to binge arose.

"Truthfully, there is a chance you will slip into that cycle again," I acknowledged. "Our eating patterns and self-esteem aren't static. You're human, and even the most disciplined humans fall back into unhealthy habits sometimes. The good news is you're more self-aware than you were a few months ago, so you'll be able to bounce back quickly."

"That is true," Josie replied thoughtfully. "I do feel more empowered than ever before."

"If you notice food has become the sole thing in your life bringing you any kind of fulfillment, you can view it as a gentle reminder there's an underlying value that needs attention," I continued. "Rather than judging yourself for eating cheese fries three days in a row because you felt lonely, acknowledge you're using it as an old coping strategy. Then, tap into your newfound strategies such as a stroll to the dog park or time with your sister to satisfy your need for connection."

"I get it," Josie said. "Instead of freaking out about what I eat and viewing it as a failure, I will choose to see it as a smoke signal. Then, I'll respond differently."

Your Turn

If or when you have another binge eating episode, revisit the root causes you identified. Then answer the following prompts:

1. Is the root cause of my binge eating emotional, physiological, or lifestyle-related?

2. How can I address or resolve this root cause?

3. Am I living in alignment with my values?

4. If not, what activities or actions can I take so I am?

Revisit these prompts regularly, making as many edits to your root causes, values, and alternative activities lists as needed. Whatever you do, don't give up! You don't need to restrict food or diet to break the binge eating cycle.

Shadow Self Integration:

- Notice how you feel or what thoughts come up before you have the urge to binge. Write down the triggers without judging yourself.

- Binging does not make you less than; it makes you human.

- Accept your strategy of using food to cope with uncomfortable feelings and triggers is no longer helpful.

- Explore which needs food is filling for you, then experiment with new activities, routines, or projects to satisfy these needs.

Chapter Takeaways

- Binge eating is not the same as overeating.

- Binge eating is a compulsive behavior that involves consuming an excessive amount of food frequently enough that it negatively impacts a person's sense of self or physical wellbeing.

- The root causes of binge eating can be physiological, lifestyle, mental, and/or emotionally-related.

- Both overexercising and dieting can lead to overeating or binge eating.

- Flow state happens when you're so immersed in a project, task, or creative pursuit that you lose track of time!

- Defining your values can help you identify how you use food to fill what's missing in your life.

- Instead of dieting or restricting, set SMART goals around new activities, routines, or projects that align with your values and put you into flow state.

- It's likely you'll fall back into unwanted eating habits now and then, and that's OK! Dust yourself off and keep moving forward!

Chapter 6

The Cardio Bunny

Shadow Tendencies:

- Exercises strictly for weight loss or burning calories

- Avoids eating before or after exercise

- Feels guilty for missing workouts

- Experiences chronic fatigue, mood swings, and cravings

- Prone to dehydration, bloat, and poor recovery

- Avoids carbohydrates and/or overeats protein during the day, but notices insatiable hunger later in the day or week

Exercise as Punishment

In the early 2000s, I grew up watching the popular TV show *America's Next Top Model*. Every afternoon, I'd come and binge watch episodes of thin women competing for the title of #1 while Tyra Banks and a panel of judges critiqued their appearance, poses, and performance. While I could go on and on about everything that was wrong with that show (such as when Lauren "Londen" Levi was kicked out of season 12 for gaining weight), my perspective on exercise was tragically altered after a single twenty-second clip from an otherwise forgettable episode.

To the camera, one of the contestants explained how she maintained her petite shape by exercising off every calorie she ate. If she ate 400 calories at lunch, she'd pedal away on the elliptical until the calorie counter ticked 400.

This made perfect sense in my undeveloped, pubescent brain. At the time, I didn't understand how the body required calories from food to function or that her behavior was disordered. Because this woman was thin—and I internalized being thin as being worthy—I thought it was *healthy*.

As a result, I developed a full-blown exercise addiction at the age of twelve. Instead of running around the neighborhood with friends after school, I did kickboxing videos in my living room. When my mom went to the YMCA after dinner, I'd tag along so I could work off the calories from dinner on the cardio machines. During 5th period Spanish, I'd fidget at my desk or pace around the classroom in an attempt to burn off lunch.

While my exercise addiction wasn't sustainable, the belief that eating was a crime punishable by hours of cardio followed me for nearly a decade. Like many All-or-Nothing Dieters, I felt *guilty* when I missed a workout. In college, I shamed myself into climbing on the Stairmaster after a meal with friends out of fear that tacos and a skinny margarita would cause me to "lose all of my progress." Not surprisingly, all of that movement made me hungrier, and because I am only human, I would eat…*a lot*.

Unlike Josie The Binge Eater who granted herself permission to eat because she exercised, I punished myself for eating by overexercising. Until I learned to fuel like an athlete, I was a **Cardio Bunny.**

Your Turn

Answer the following questions. Do you...

1. Exercise with the primary goal of burning calories for weight loss?

2. Feel guilty for eating before or after exercise?

3. Beat yourself up for missing a workout?

4. Tack on extra cardio the day(s) following a heavier meal?

5. Assume a workout is a waste if you didn't sweat or elevate your heart rate?

6. Think a training session is incomplete without cardio?

7. Set goals around how many calories you burn during exercise?

8. Workout consistently for short periods followed by stretches of inactivity or burn out?

9. Experience chronic fatigue, mood swings, and cravings?

10. Eat plenty of protein during the day but experience cravings for carbohydrates or sugar?

11. Have trouble recovering from tough workouts?

If you answered "yes" to three or more of these questions, you may identify with shadow tendencies of The Cardio Bunny sub-archetype. The strategies in this chapter will help you manage your relationship to food and exercise.

Fuel Like an Athlete

Cardio Bunnies are conditioned to eat less and move more to lose weight, which is detrimental to their progress, metabolism, and mental wellbeing. Not eating enough calories to match activity levels also increases the risk of injury and prolongs existing ones.

On the flip side, mindlessly eating junk or greasy snacks before a workout is also a recipe for disaster. Who wants to put in all that work just to feel sluggish or tired?

The middle ground is learning to fuel like an athlete. Just like Venus Williams wouldn't skip meals before training, recreational athletes need fuel to get the most out of their workouts.

It's not just team sports players who benefit from fueling like an athlete but anyone who trains! Examples of athletes include…

- Group fitness junkies (HIIT or barre classes)

- Pilates enthusiasts and yogis

- Dancers and cheerleaders

- Bodybuilders and powerlifters

- Crossfitters

- Endurance athletes (cycling, running, swimming)

- Power athletes (rowing, sprinting, gymnasts)

- Wrestlers and mixed martial artists

- Peloton and cycle studio fanatics

Heck, even dog walkers are athletes in my book. No matter their skill level, my active clients who think of themselves as athletes begin to reframe how they fuel their body. This encourages them to take care of their physical bodies with proper sleep, hydration, recovery, and of course, food. Prioritizing nutrition requires understanding how to eat, planning ahead, and commitment to fueling.

Your Turn

If you are able-bodied and not engaging in regular physical activity, it's time to commit to moving your body. Pick something you enjoy (or think you'd enjoy) and schedule it at least twice this week.

Running on Empty

Athletes eat a healthy diet, but they *do not* diet. This was news for my client Aniyah, a 39-year-old marathon runner, full-time mother, and part-time dieter. She was referred to me by her running coach to improve her performance at races, reduce bloat, and lose the baby weight from eight years ago.

"Hi," I greeted her as she poked her head in the door, unsure if she was in the right place. "Are you Aniyah?"

"That's me!" she said as she stepped forward.

Aniyah was one of those women who was so gorgeous you wanted to hate her, but her fun-loving and kind personality made it impossible not to adore her! Her 5'8" frame was all legs and her dark chocolate-colored skin perfectly complimented her light brown eyes and sparkly white teeth. The first day we met, she wore her black hair in a braided top bun and sported a matching violet workout tank and shorts.

"That's a cute outfit," I complimented, genuinely impressed by the fact that she looked so comfy yet chic. "Where's it from?"

"Thank you! Believe it or not, Amazon," Aniyah replied. "It's a dupe of one of those high-end athleisure brands, but it looks just as good for a third of the price."

A woman who doesn't gatekeep[22]? I liked her already.

After we got acquainted, I asked Aniyah how she felt about being referred to a registered dietitian. From my experience, the most successful clients are the ones who actually want to be in my office and aren't speaking with me out of obligation.

---

[22] *Gatekeep (v): the act of controlling, and usually limiting, general access to something.*

Luckily, Aniyah appeared to be there on her own will.

"I'm equal parts excited and nervous," she confessed. "Before my coach suggested I come here, I never thought about talking to someone about how I ate. I started running two years ago after my divorce because I was motivated to get back to my pre-pregnancy weight. Running is such a great way for me to burn off stress, but lately I am dragging through my workouts. I refuse to believe it's because I am turning forty this year, so it's gotta be the food."

After she confirmed she had no recent injuries, vitamin and mineral deficiencies, or difficulty sleeping, I asked her to rate her current energy on a scale of 1-10 before and after her runs.

"On my best days, I start at six or seven but end between two and four," Aniyah said. "I'm totally wiped! I'd like to finish my workout feeling more energized than when I started."

"What's a normal day of eating and training look like for you?"

"I wrote it down for you." Aniyah reached into her purse and pulled out neatly folded papers. Pinned to her bag's handle were at least a dozen pins from Disney World.

Working in Orlando, the theme park capital of the world, meant a lot of my clients participated in races hosted by "The Most Magical Place on Earth." While some ran solely for the fun of dressing up as their favorite characters and collecting medals, others signed up to beat personal records and place high in their age groups.

"I'm currently training for the Dopey Challenge in January," Aniyah replied as she handed me her food and exercise notes. "I'll be running their 5k on Thursday, a 10k on Friday, a half marathon on Saturday, and a full marathon on Sunday."

My jaw dropped. Did I hear her correctly?

"Yeah, it's intense." Aniyah read my expression and giggled. "A total of forty-eight-point-six miles in four days. Go big or go home, right?"

"That's what they say," I laughed half-heartedly. As someone who stresses about jogging an occasional 5k for charity, I couldn't understand how someone would willingly sign themselves up for an entire weekend of non-stop foot-to-pavement. She must be psycho, and I loved it.

"Let's take a look at how you're fueling for this torture, I mean, *adventure*."

Aniyah's Current Meal Plan

Time	Meal
Pre-Run Meal	Low-carb protein bar
Post-Run Meal	Egg white omelet with veggies and ¼ avocado One small nectarine
Lunch	Green salad with grilled chicken, cheese, cucumbers, and low-calorie vinaigrette
Snack 1	Non-fat, sugar-free Greek yogurt mixed with peanut butter powder
Snack 2	Low-carb protein bar
Dinner	Grilled chicken, steak, or salmon with a veggie salad
Dessert	Handful of almonds and cup of blueberries

Table 2.6.1

To The All-or-Nothing Dieter, Aniyah's high protein and low-carb meal plan[23] might look like the pinnacle of health. But this ain't my first rodeo with so-called "low-carb" athletes, and I suspected she was only sharing the highlight reel rather than the whole story.

"If this is how you really ate and it was working for you, you wouldn't be in my office today," I pointed out after reviewing her diet recall. "Can I take a stab and guess this recount of your average day of eating is more of what you try to follow rather than what you *actually* do?"

"Ha, busted," Aniyah said, her cheeks turning a slight shade of pink.

"Let's talk about what's really going on," I said, crumpling her meal plan and tossing it aside.

"I don't know what's wrong with me," Aniyah huffed. "I feel like I am eating all day but once I begin to cook dinner, I feel ravenous. I

---

[23] *There is no fixed definition for a low-carb diet. In this book, a low-carb diet is defined as a purposeful restriction of carbohydrate to less than 30% of one's total diet.*

start to pick at my son's snacks, potato chips and sour candy. After we eat, I still find myself snacking on whatever I can find."

"More candy and chips?" I asked.

"No, that'd at least be somewhat normal," she replied. "Nothing I eat after dinner makes sense. I'll melt handfuls of chocolate chips with butter and scoop it out with graham crackers or dip carrots in crunchy peanut butter. If I don't have many groceries, I'll eat two or three of my low-carb protein bars with hazelnut spread melted on top."

As a result of her late-night eating, Aniyah often woke up early for her morning runs and wondered why she literally *had* the runs.

"I call it my poop loop," Aniyah laughed. "I'll make it about two miles before I have to stop and crap my pants. Not only do I experience painful bloating, all of the stop and go is interfering with my training. I need help!"

The issue was clear: Aniyah was not eating nearly enough carbohydrates before, during, and after her runs. As a result, she was overeating large quantities of dietary fat, sugar, and protein bars with sugar alcohols. The following day, her digestive tract paid the price.

Clearly, a low-carb diet high in ultra-processed supplements was not working for Aniyah's body or training routine. I wanted her to consider if adding in whole foods, including carbohydrates, would help her feel and perform at her best.

"I saw on your appointment notes that you have a son," I said, deciding to make my point personal. "Does he play sports?"

"He just started playing little league baseball." She flashed me her phone home screen, a picture of her crouching next to her son in his helmet and uniform. "His name is Jackson, named after my father."

"Jackson is a cutie!" I gushed. "What do you feed him to fuel for games and practice?"

"Lately, he's been asking for peanut butter and banana sandwiches. If he just needs a snack, I will fix him a fruit platter with almonds and crackers. Jackson also *loves* oatmeal. I joke that he's a little old man because what eight-year-old asks for oatmeal?"

"One who has a mom who serves him healthy foods," I smiled. "Specifically, healthy carbohydrates. It's interesting how you gladly serve Jackson the fuel he needs to run and play but deprive yourself of the same foods."

Aniyah looked rather taken aback. After a moment, she told me, "I never thought of it that way. I'm terrified of eating too many carbs. I'm afraid they'll make me fat."

When I asked Aniyah how often she weighed herself, she told me almost daily.

"I hate the scale and the power it has over me," she admitted. "Even just a one-pound increase can put me out of a good mood."

The Scale Sucks

While the scale can be a helpful tool for measuring progress over a long period of time, it's not a useful tool for day-to-day progress. This is because weight fluctuates as you eat, drink, breathe, poop, sweat, and urinate throughout a 24-hour period.

If you have had the experience of gaining weight after a so-called "perfect day" of exercising and eating, the scale going up can feel frustrating and make you want to give up completely. However, there are at least nine reasons the scale ticked up:

Water Intake: This may be the most obvious reason why the scale fluctuates, but what actually influences fluid shifts in our body besides drinking and sweating? Salt and glycogen cause our bodies to temporarily hold onto water while caffeine, alcohol, and diuretics make us sweat or pee out fluids.

Sodium: Dietary sodium is crucial for health, especially if you're exercising and/or working outdoors. However, water follows salt, which explains why you may feel bloated or notice a weight increase after dining out. Even if you ordered something healthy, restaurants typically use a lot more salt in their cooking. Does this mean you should never eat out? Absolutely not! Just don't get freaked out by a slight increase in weight the day after. Balance it out by eating whole, minimally processed foods for the rest of the day and drinking plenty of fluid.

Sleep: Ever notice how you weigh less on Sunday morning, even when you've indulged a bit on Saturday? Many people use weekends to sleep in, giving the body extra time to shift fluid from cells to the bloodstream. From there, fluid is sent to our kidneys so it can be excreted when we urinate the next morning. Therefore, we're losing additional ounces in water weight.

Fiber: Many of my clients feel discouraged when they notice water retention after increasing their vegetable and fiber intake. Fiber is indigestible and introducing large amounts at one time may make you feel bloated. Since fiber is a key component for weight loss, blood sugar stability, heart, and digestive health, don't let initial water weight keep you from eating it. Your body will adjust as you increase and maintain fiber intake. Be sure to drink extra water to help move things along!

Glycogen: Glycogen is stored energy from carbohydrates. For every gram of glycogen stored, our bodies retain 2-3 grams of water! This can explain why people who follow a ketogenic or very low-carb eating plan may experience rapid weight loss in the initial phases of the diet. Your body holds on to this water for good reasons. A well-hydrated muscle tissue is a healthy tissue. Water transports vital nutrients to the cells to aid in cellular functions such as muscle synthesis. So don't fret if you notice the scale jump days after a high carb meal. It's likely not related to body fat, it's just part of how your body utilizes carbohydrates.

Inflammation & Muscle Soreness: Ever crush a workout only to be dismantled by a weight increase the following day? Exercise breaks down muscle tissue, sending the signal to your body there is damage. Therefore, it holds water and targets inflamed tissues to help heal and soothe swelling. In case you need another reason to wear sunscreen, this explains why a sunburn can cause water retention.

Hormonal Shifts: Many women experience water retention about a week before their menstrual cycle due to increase of sex hormones progesterone and estrogen. Two to five pounds of weight gain during this time is to be expected. Don't panic, things will settle back to baseline after your period. If you struggle with bloat before your period, a low sodium diet, adequate fiber, and plenty of water can help ease the symptoms.

Muscle Growth: One exciting reason the scale isn't dropping may be due to an increase in lean muscle mass, particularly if you are exercising regularly. While this shift is not instantaneous, muscle growth slows weight loss but improves your physique and boosts your metabolism.

Creatine: The supplement creatine can cause 'intra-cellular' water retention, meaning it is stored within the cell itself rather than underneath the skin. This explains the weight gained after taking a creatine supplement, even though you may not experience any side effects such as abdominal bloating.

Monitoring Weight Changes

If you choose to use the scale to monitor weight loss, weigh under consistent conditions (i.e, same scale, time, clothes, empty bladder), record your weight 4-7x per week and average those numbers. Tracking your weekly average weight will identify a trend. More than 1% body weight lost in one week is likely influenced by water. If you notice the scale is negatively impacting your behaviors around food, lock that thing up and throw away the key.

Better ways to measure progress include:

Getting a DexaScan

Measuring body parts including arm, thigh, waist, and/or hip

Snapping progress pictures

Rating your energy levels on a scale from 1-10

Rating your mood on a scale from 1-10

Be sure to make notes about which day of your menstrual cycle you are measuring, as hormonal shifts throughout your cycle influence outcomes.

Carbs are Fuel

"I heard you say you're turning forty this year," I said, switching gears. "Are you anxious about it?"

"Me? Hell no!" Aniyah belly-laughed and playfully shook her finger. "After the all the crap I went through in my thirties, I say bring it. It's going to be the best decade of me and Jackson's life!"

Aniyah told me after her mother-in-law passed away during the pandemic, her once doting husband Jose began neglecting their marriage because he was too busy putting his lips to a bottle. Refusing to go to therapy or face his grief in healthy ways, his drinking problem got worse and worse. Prior to his mother's death, Jose had been the type to order an innocent lemonade with lunch or tea with dinner. But he began replacing meals altogether with booze, and booze made him angry.

"We'd been together for six years, and I had never seen Jose even raise his voice," Aniyah recalled. "He was gentle and reserved, the perfect balance to my loud and in-your-face energy. I kept hoping he'd snap back to normal, but I was naive. After I found a half empty vodka bottle hidden in Jackson's laundry basket, things escalated. He threw his family's gold Asprey bird statue at the wall behind me, and I told him he needed to get the hell out of my house."

My eyes widened. "Aren't those like…"

"Hundreds of thousands of dollars?" Aniyah finished my thought. "Mm-hmm. But it's only money. Better him to break a statue than to lay a hand on me and our son."

I didn't know how to react, so I sat silently in complete awe of this woman's strength. Aniyah had lost not only her mother-in-law during a global pandemic but the father of her son. Yet here she was, a single mom who protected her baby, ran marathons, and was determined to have the best, healthiest year of her life. I was honored to be on her team.

"I'm so sorry you went through all of that," I finally mustered, though my words didn't do her story justice.

Through a warm smile she said, "Thank you. But I'm not here to dwell on the past. I'm here to crush this race and look good doing it!"

With that, I remembered why I brought up her age in the first place. "Do you have any fears or insecurities about your body changing in your forties?"

"Don't we all? It seems like with every passing decade, I gain ten pounds."

"Do you think a low-carb diet will help you lose weight?" I asked.

"Worked for me in the past. Before vacations, weddings, or special events, I'd cut out bread, pasta, and potatoes and drop weight like that." Aniyah snapped her fingers.

"Were you exercising then?"

She shook her head no, stating she had worked as an attorney who barely had time to leave her desk for a water break.

It was starting to make sense. Aniyah was avoiding carbs because she was afraid of gaining weight, so she employed old tricks to help her shed a few pounds. But as her body changed with age and her activity level skyrocketed, she needed to adapt to a sustainable approach that *wouldn't* cause her to poop her pants. Aniyah needed to understand how carbohydrates were her friend, not foe.

"Unlike fat and protein, carbohydrates are quickly converted into energy for our bodies to use as fuel," I explained. "Without enough carbs, our body has to rely on less efficient sources of fuel for energy. This leads to poor performance, muscle loss, fatigue, lack of motivation and focus, mood swings, digestive distress, and intense cravings for sugar."

Aniyah recited the side effects while counting the pads of her fingers. "Poor performance, fatigue, digestive issues, and cravings... Yep, I've got 'em all."

"Given your diet, that checks," I assured her. "Whether your goal is fat loss, better performance, or simply to feel *good*, you'll benefit from consuming carbohydrates throughout the day. You'll have better workouts and won't feel like passing out after a session."

"Or passing through a Krispy Kreme drive-thru on the way home," Aniyah laughed. "But in all seriousness, won't eating too many carbs make me fat?"

"No, carbs won't make you fat," I said. "Weight gain is a lot more complicated than eating too many bananas and potatoes."

"Bananas are sugar sticks," Aniyah said, almost reflexively. She had caught the diet culture bug, and she had it *bad*.

"If diet culture has made you too scared to eat whole food sources of carbohydrates like bananas, consider how many foods contain carbs," I said, handing her the list of complex carbs from the BNT Protocol. "Avoiding vegetables, starches, fruits, beans, legumes, dairy, oats, and grains means avoiding *most* food. On their own, these foods are perfectly nutritious and difficult to overeat because they contain fiber."

"And without seasoning, most of these foods are bland!" Aniyah scrunched her nose.

"Eh, agree to disagree," I said. "Carbohydrate-rich foods like caramel lattes, BBQ potato chips, and cream cheese bagels are easy to overeat because they're *hyperpalatable*. This means they're higher in calories or sugar, low in fiber, and processed to improve texture or flavor."

"So you're saving the hyperpalatable foods that contain carbohydrates are the ones giving *all* carbs a bad rep?" Aniyah asked.

"Yes and no," I answered. "No foods are bad, but some are easier to overeat and don't provide much nutritional benefit. Eating carbohydrates with added fats from oils or cheese can also make you feel sluggish before a run. This is why choosing complex carbs over refined options and spacing them throughout the day will fuel powerful workouts, help you fill up on less food, and regulate your digestion."

Your Turn

Have you ever followed low-carb diets such as Atkins, Keto, or a macro-counting approach where less than 30% of your total food intake came from carbohydrates? If so, answer the following prompts comparing a low-carb diet to a balanced diet per the BNT Protocol.

On a low-carb diet, did my..

- ...motivation to be active increase, decrease, or stay the same?

- ...energy levels increase, decrease, or stay the same?

- ...cravings increase, decrease, or stay the same?

- ...mood increase, decrease, or stay the same?

- ...stamina, endurance, and/or strength increase, decrease, or stay the same?

- ...digestion improve, worsen, or stay the same?

- **Optional:** If you were purposefully trying to lose weight during a low-carb diet, did your weight increase, decrease, or stay the same? If it decreased, were you able to sustain the loss?

Reflect on your answers. If you saw a decrease in motivation, energy, cravings, mood, stamina, was it worth it?

How about digestive distress? If weight loss was not sustainable, was it because of these side effects?

Eating Protein Like a Bodybuilder

Protein is required to build muscle tissue, which comes with many benefits including fat loss and increased metabolism. However, many women mistakenly believe they should be eating more than one gram of protein per pound of their goal body weight (or current weight) to tone up and lose weight.Usually this is because an online fitness influencer or bodybuilder recommended it.

Many bodybuilders *do* eat that much protein...with equal or twice as many total carbohydrates! They know the body's top priority is to keep them alive, and the glucose from carbohydrates provides ready-to-use energy that keeps their body functioning well. Unlike carbohydrates, protein is **not** a good source of energy. When the body does not receive enough energy, it converts protein into energy as a last resort.

This is **not** good. Instead of using amino acids from protein to build fat-burning muscle, they're doing what carbohydrates could have done better.

Bodybuilders decrease total carbs only after they've spent a lot of time and sweat in the gym building lean muscle. Because they **are literally starving themselves**, their protein intake must remain high so they don't lose precious muscle tissue as their body eats itself. Once they've reached an unsustainable body fat percentage for show day, they return to eating carbohydrates and regain any weight they lost.

The rest of us should not be starving ourselves to lose weight. Instead, women who want to tone-up and reshape their body benefit from both patience *and* eating complex carbs with their protein.

Fueling on Fat?

"What do you think about the keto diet everyone's talking about?" Aniyah asked. She was referring to the ketogenic diet (mentioned in the Fundamentals of Balanced Nutrition).

"I think it'll amplify your poop loop," my tone was playful, but I was dead serious.

"For real?"

"Too much dietary fat can cause your colon to overproduce liquid, leading to loose stools or diarrhea," I explained. "Fiber from complex carbs helps bind food in your gut, which makes for way more comfortable bowel movements."

"Yikes," Aniyah said. "I may have that problem now."

"Do you also experience bloat, pain, or distention of your gut?"

She nodded her head vigorously.

"That could also be a side effect of too much dietary fat. I noticed your pre-run snack is a low-carb protein bar. These are often high in dietary fats, which is not recommended before physical activity."

I went on to explain that while the calories from dietary fat and carbohydrates can be used for energy, it takes the body longer to break down fat and turn it into fuel. Fats, even the healthy ones, sit in the stomach longer than carbohydrates.

"This is why the idea of eating avocado and oily eggs right before exercise may make you want to throw up," I mentioned. "Dietary fat should *not* make up the majority of calories for an active person. Instead, aim for a fourth or a third of your diet to come from healthy fats. Spread your intake evenly throughout the day, eating slightly less right before vigorous activity to prevent digestive distress."

A Note on Bloat

After a day of eating, it's normal for your stomach to expand with food, air, and fluid. That is not bloat. Bloating is abnormal and is marked by having gas, a hard or distended abdomen, and pressure or tightness in the gut.

Common causes of bloat include:

- Ingesting foods or supplements that contain sugar alcohols (erythritol, maltitol, mannitol, sorbitol, xylitol)

- Consuming large quantities of sugar-free gum, candies, or mints

- Eating an excess of high-fiber vegetables, specifically uncooked cruciferous veggies like broccoli, kale, Brussels sprouts, cauliflower, and bok choy

- Drinking carbonated beverages

- Drinking through a straw

- Lactose intolerance, specifically from milk or ice cream

- Dehydration

More extreme causes include food sensitivities such as Celiac disease, gluten intolerance, small intestinal bacterial overgrowth (SIBO), or having difficulty digesting foods that contain FODMAPS such as garlic or onion. FODMAP stands for fermentable oligosaccharides, disaccharides, monosaccharides and polyols, which are short-chain carbohydrates that the small intestine absorbs poorly. Meet with a registered dietitian to manage symptoms.

Pre-Workout Nutrition

"So what *should* I be eating before a run to ensure I'm comfortable?" Aniyah asked.

"First, avoid anything too high in fat as that may make you feel sluggish," I said, referring to the BNT Protocol's list of healthy fats. "This takes trial and error. A spoonful of peanut butter with a banana may be comfortable for me but it may not sit as well with you."

I showed her a list of other fat containing foods I do not recommend pre-workout:

- Greasy food like French fries, burgers, and pizza

- Spicy foods

- Full-fat dairy from cheese, yogurt, cottage cheese, and milk

- Nuts and seeds

"Do people really eat fast food before a workout?" Aniyah remarked, arching her brow as she looked over the short list.

"You'd be surprised," I answered. I thought of my client Joel, who would eat a Burger King Whopper before hopping on his bike in the hot Florida sun. He wondered why he bonked[24] after just seven miles.

"I am surprised nuts are on this list, though," Aniyah admitted. "Aren't they healthy?"

"Yes, but healthy doesn't mean they're a good source of fuel for exercise," I said. "Since they're higher in healthy fats and low in carbohydrates, you'd only want a small portion of nuts paired with a source of carbs, such as fruit or toast. "Before a workout, your body needs easy-to-digest carbohydrates to fuel your activity. Carbs too high in fiber, such as unripe fruit or fiber-enhanced cereals, can cause digestive issues. With both fat and fiber, it takes some trial and error to learn what works for you, but here are some ideas to help you plan your pre-exercise meals."

---

[24] *Bonking is the shut down of all body systems during exercise. It occurs when the muscles become functionally depleted of glycogen, the carbohydrate energy stores by which the body fuels itself.*

I handed Aniyah two charts, the first comparing the best pre-workout snacks to eat within an hour of exercise.

Fueling 20 to 60 Minutes Before a Workout

Instead of...	Try...
Fibrous fruit such as unripe bananas or apples	Ripe banana with smear of natural nut butter
A large smoothie with full-fat yogurt, chia seeds, nut butter, and fruit	Fruit smoothie with scoop of whey protein
Avocado toast with a fried egg	Toast with hard-boiled egg
Protein shake in almond milk or water	Protein shake with oat milk or skim milk
Nut mix	Orange slices with a small handful of almonds
Low-carb protein bars	Whole food energy bar with at least 20 grams of carbohydrate

Table 2.6.2

The second chart gave examples of complete meals to eat within one to three hours of exercise.

"Most people can tolerate fat and fiber in their diet an hour before exercise," I explained. "The body has more time to break down and digest these foods. Eating complex carbs and protein should remain a priority."

Fueling 1 to 3 Hours Before a Workout

Instead of...	Try...
Salad with grilled chicken, pecans, and balsamic vinaigrette	Salad with grilled chicken, pecans, a scoop of quinoa, strawberry slices, and balsamic vinaigrette
Tilapia and broccoli	Salmon, sweet potato, and broccoli
Chocolate keto bomb	Dark chocolate square with cherries
Fried rice with crispy tofu and a Coke	Brown rice with baked tofu, fresh pineapple chunks, carrots sticks, and mineral water
Tortilla chips and guacamole	Hummus with whole grain pita bread and carrot sticks

Table 2.6.3

"I don't recommend doing intense exercise on an empty stomach," I told Aniyah. "A light walk or jog may be fine, but don't train on E. If you don't have an appetite, try a homemade sports drink, sports gel, chew, or salted medjool date to get you through the run."

Your Turn

If you experience digestive distress and bloat around or during exercise, take a look at your pre-workout fuel. Is there too much dietary fat? Or difficult-to-digest fiber?

Using Table 2.6.2, brainstorm two ideas for pre-workout fuel within an hour of exercise.

Using Table 2.6.3, brainstorm two ideas for pre-workout fuel 1-3 hours before exercise.

Intra-Workout Fuel

"Now that we've planned pre-workout fuel, let's talk about what to eat during a workout," I said. "Athletes who exercise for one hour or more or for at least forty-five minutes at a high intensity require intra-workout glucose to keep going. Otherwise, the body runs out of fuel and performance suffers. Recreational athletes exercising less than an hour do not need intra-workout glucose."

"My running coach has me eating sports gels and sports beans during runs. Are those okay?" asked Aniyah.

"Sports beans, gels, chews, and natural drinks provide quick sources of carbohydrate, making them great for intra-workout fuel," I replied. "They're easy to digest and travel well during runs, bike rides, games, or gym sessions. Dried fruit like raisins or salted medjool dates are also fan favorites."

"Okay, but I'm not clear on when or how much to eat."

"At the forty-five to sixty-minute mark, ingest at least fifteen to thirty grams of quick-digesting glucose from natural sports drinks, powders, gels, beans, or dried fruit. Check the nutrition label to determine how many grams of carbs are in a serving. For instance, a Honey Stinger sports gel has about twenty-four grams of carbs, making one packet a solid choice. Then, repeat this serving every fifteen to thirty minutes," I said. "Doing so may help you end your runs on a high note and help you hit personal records."

"What about when I strength train?" Aniyah said. "I lift for about an hour, but I am taking breaks to rest in between exercise sets."

"If you are resting between sets, you do not need to fuel during lifts," I answered. "Hydrate with water and prioritize pre- and post-workout nutrition."

Your Turn

If you are exercising for an hour or more OR for 45 minutes at a high intensity, circle which intra-workout options sound appealing:

- Natural sports drink

- Sports chew, gel, or bean

- Sports honey waffle

- Dried fruit

- Honey or maple syrup

Post-Workout Nutrition & Timing

"I know protein is important for recovery, which is why I usually eat my egg white omelet after training or running," Aniyah said. "Sometimes I'll add turkey bacon for an extra boost."

Aniyah was right. Consuming at least 20-40 grams of protein is beneficial at all meals but especially post-exercise as it helps build and recover muscle tissue broken down during training. It also helps with satiety and prevents blood sugar crashes, which makes eating a balanced, portion-controlled diet much easier.

"Forty grams seems like a lot," Aniyah commented.

Even though Aniyah's current meal plan had her eating the recommended amount of protein per meal, I showed her a list of meals that contain 20-40 grams of protein.

20-40 grams of protein looks like....

Meal	Total Protein
2 eggs scrambled with ¼ cup cheese and slice of sprouted grain toast	22 grams
1 cup of plain, 2% Greek yogurt with a tablespoon of nuts and berries	23 grams
4 ounces tempeh with brown rice, ¼ cup cashews, and stir-fried veggies	26 grams
4 ounces of chicken breast with ½ cup beans, salsa, and roasted veggies	35 grams
1 slice Ezekiel bread with 3 ounces salmon lox and 1 tablespoon cream cheese	23 grams
3 ounce turkey patty with 1 slice of cheese, tomato, and whole wheat bun	39 grams

Table 2.6.4

"Since I need to eat carbohydrates before I workout, do I need to eat them after?" Aniyah asked.

"Yep," I replied. "After exhausting your body from workouts, you need to refuel with plenty of carbohydrates. This helps replenish the energy stores drained during exercise. Remember, without enough carbs, your body will convert protein to energy instead of recovering muscle tissue."

"I have a small nectarine with my post-workout egg white omelet. Is that enough?" Aniyah asked.

I shot her a look that said, *Not even close, honey.* "You'll need *the same or up to three times as many* carbohydrates as protein post-workout. This means one puny nectarine won't cut it."

Looking puzzled, Aniyah whipped out her phone and began frantically tapping her fingers on the keyboard. Without glancing up, she said, "Looks like there are fifteen grams of carbohydrate in a nectarine, so I could eat two for thirty grams. That'd be the same or slightly more protein than I'm eating."

I nodded. "Yep, but you have room for more if you notice you're still struggling with cravings, hunger, or poor recovery. In that case, you could add a serving of old-fashioned oats or a slice of toast."

While I wanted Aniyah to understand the science behind post-workout nutrition, I did not want her to get bogged down by the numbers. What mattered was that she follow the BNT Protocol with an emphasis on carbs and protein post-workout.

"Oatmeal?" Aniyah playfully stuck out her tongue in disgust. "I'll save that mush for Jackson. What about a strawberry Toaster Strudel? I have been jonesing for one lately!"

"Only if you're okay with a sugar crash later," I grinned. "Plus, I want you to eat more fiber to improve your digestion. Let me show you some healthy alternatives to post-workout meals."

Post-Workout Meals and Snacks Ideas

Instead of This...	...Try This!
Water	Chocolate milk and water (separate, of course!)
A protein shake blended with water	A scoop of protein blended with frozen fruit with any unsweetened milk of your choice
Breaded nuggets with ranch sauce, fries, and lemonade	Grilled chicken in a whole grain wrap with a fruit cup and water
Low-carb protein bar with iced almond milk latte	RxBar with soy, oat, or cow's milk latte
Egg white omelet with cheese and turkey bacon	2 egg pasture-raised egg omelet with veggies and cheese with side of sprouted grain toast
Sugary cereal with almond milk	Overnight oats made with protein powder and unsweetened milk of choice, topped with fruit
Teriyaki stir-fry with veggies, cauliflower rice, and cashews	Teriyaki stir-fry with veggies, quinoa, cashews, and extra firm tofu
Nothing	Something

Table 2.6.5

Aniyah pointed her finger to the last row, commenting that she is often not hungry right after a long run. "Should I force myself to eat?"

"Nope," I reassured her. "Having a suppressed appetite after exercise is normal. Practice mindfulness and check in with your body periodically. If you wait more than four hours after your last meal, you may experience a crash."

"I thought your B-N- *whatever* protocol said to eat every three to six hours?" Aniyah said. "Why within four hours?"

"When you're exercising, your body is burning through energy at a faster rate than it would if you were sitting at your desk or on a road trip. This means you'll need to refuel sooner rather than later," I said.

"So if I eat lunch at 1 p.m. and finish exercising at 3 PM, I should eat no later than 5 PM?"

"Exactly," I affirmed. "Eat right before you begin to feel hungry. Do not stave off hunger in an effort to 'save calories' or finish a task."

Aniyah looked worried, and I asked what she was thinking.

"I'm hesitant to increase my carbohydrates during the day," she admitted, shaking her head back and forth. "I don't trust myself not to overeat at night, and I'm afraid all of this eating will make me gain weight. I wish I wasn't such a food addict."

Aniyah was not a food addict. She was simply undereating, causing her to *feel* like an addict around hyperpalatable foods at night.

Your Turn

Do you feel addicted to sugar or hyperpalatable foods like chips, pizza, or French fries? If so, could it be because you're eating an imbalance of the right nutrients, skipping meals, or underfueling for exercise?

Is Food Addictive?

The American Journal of Nutrition released a Great Debates in Nutrition consensus paper in 2021 to evaluate arguments on whether or not highly processed foods have addictive potential. If you're familiar with reading research papers, you know they end with "more evidence is needed," and this study was no exception. There are still too many gaps in the research and undecided criteria needed to resolve the debate on whether food is an addictive substance like tobacco, or if it should be included in the Diagnostic and Statistical Manual of Mental Disorders, Edition 5 (DSM-5) category "Substance-related and addictive disorders."

However, both sides of the argument had a few points of agreement, including that there are eating behaviors consistent with the phenotype of a so-called food addict. These behaviors included:

- Having little control over how much or what they consume

- Reporting intense cravings

- Overconsumption of food despite unwanted side effects (physical discomfort, weight gain, digestive issues, diet-related diseases)

- Repeated failed attempts to better control eating behaviors

The report noted that obese individuals have a higher prevalence of addictive eating habits, but people of any weight can regularly engage in these behaviors. Both sides also agreed The Yale Food Addiction Scale, which ranks the frequency of addictive-like food behaviors, is useful for assessing behaviors around food. If you're curious about this scale, you can find it with an easy Google search. Although I acknowledge hyperpalatable foods may feel addictive, I've noticed my clients who call themselves food addicts are also consuming an imbalance of nutrients. They skip breakfast or don't fuel up with protein, fiber, or complex carbohydrates, then wonder why they can't stop munching on Chex Mix after dinner. Once they start following The BNT Protocol, addictive-like tendencies around food slow down dramatically.

Dopamine Junkie

"I do think you have some habits around eating that make you *feel* addicted to food, but I would not label you as a food addict," I told Aniyah. "You're just stuck in a cycle of restrictive eating."

For All-or-Nothing dieters, restricting and binging food feels addicting because it offers a hit of dopamine. Dopamine is the chemical messenger responsible for driving behaviors that offer a desired outcome or pleasure response. It's a part of the "reward system" in our brain which encourages people to repeat actions that feel good or provide a sense of enjoyment. Binge eating activates the same dopamine response as alcohol or drug use and explains why it feels addicting.

In my experience, I've noticed All-or-Nothing dieters not only derive pleasure from sneak eating, emotional eating, or binge eating but also dieting behaviors. Stepping on the scale and seeing the number decrease feels rewarding, encouraging a dieter to continue restrictive behaviors. On the flip side, seeing undesired results can make her feel crummy. As a means to feel better instantly, she eats or restricts.

"Dieting *does* feel addictive," Aniyah exclaimed. "I feel a rewarding rush when I follow my meal plan to a T. I feel so accomplished, as if I checked off an important task on my to-do list. Plus, it feels great to see my weight drop after I crushed the day. Is that bad?"

"Not necessarily," I said. "But your brain begins to associate food restriction with the reward of quick weight loss when the two might not be related. This motivates you to continue dieting, even if you can't keep it up for more than a few days. After you overeat and regain the weight, your brain will motivate you to seek out a reward the only way it knows how—dieting."

"So the reason I overeat at night is mental and physical," Aniyah said thoughtfully. "Not only am I not eating enough to meet my basic needs, but I am motivated to lose weight. I've trained myself to quickly get that reward by under-eating until that backfires. Then, I get my next dopamine fix by eating a bunch of sugary and ultra-processed foods at night."

"You're getting it!" I balled my hands into loose fists, set them on my desk, and leaned forward. "Not only does eating release dopamine, so does the mere anticipation of food. Imagine sitting in a restaurant and seeing the waiter walking over with your meal. It's the most exciting feeling ever, right?"

Aniyah laughed and nodded.

"The dopamine release motivates you to waste no time picking up your fork and chowing down," I explained. "But with each consecutive bite, the dopamine response diminishes. This is why the first bite of pasta tastes so much better than the fourth or fifth. People who consistently fuel throughout the day are more aware of this and have an easier time stopping once they are satisfied. But when your body is malnourished, stopping feels impossible."

"I think I had this experience the other day after my nine-mile run," Aniyah replied. "I ate two meals, but I couldn't stop thinking about my son's cheese puffs in the pantry. I don't even like the way they taste, but I couldn't stop eating them once I started. After I had my fun, I felt miserable. That is, until I started thinking about the big jar of unopened peanut butter…"

Aniyah had cracked the code. Starving her body during the day resulted in overeating junk food, which negatively impacted her workouts, digestion, and weight loss goals.

Your Turn

Are you addicted to dieting? Reflect on your own restrictive-eating behaviors that give you a dopamine hit. Dieting behaviors that feel rewarding include:

- Tracking food in a digital app
- Meeting restrictive calorie or macronutrient goals
- Measuring food on a food scale
- Skipping meals
- Obsessive weighing on the scale

- Crossing off diet behaviors on a to-do list (i.e, *drank 1 gallon of water, did not eat carbs at dinner*)

- Overexercising

Are any of these behaviors causing negative side effects?

Pain Before Pleasure

Paul Bloom states in his book *The Sweet Spot: The Pleasures of Suffering and the Search for Meaning*, "the simplest theory of human nature is that we work like hell to avoid pain. We pursue pleasure and comfort; we hope to make it through life unscathed. Suffering and pain are by their very nature, to be avoided... but this theory is incomplete. Under the right circumstances and in the right doses, physical pain and emotional pain, difficulty and failure and loss, are exactly what we are looking for."

Essentially, he's saying humans have it all wrong when it comes to happiness. We think more pleasure means less pain, when it's actually the other way around. Rather, we derive more life and personal satisfaction when we WILLINGLY pursue self-induced suffering. Of course this does not include suffering in the form of torture, trauma, accidents, or death. Purposely seeking challenges such as lifting weights, taking a cold shower, or spending a hot afternoon digging in a garden leaves us feeling fulfilled while watching TikTok all day feels like crap. Even though an occasional lazy afternoon is necessary, too many days of being a bum leaves us craving something more — more sugar, more UberEats, more *dopamine hits*.

Spend the day accomplishing difficult things and notice how you feel afterwards. Curling up at night with your phone is much more rewarding after working on a meaningful project or prepping food for the week. Your baseline level of satisfaction is higher, and therefore your need for more pleasure from food is less intense.

I tell my clients they can choose their suffering. Either give into instant gratification and deal with consequences later, or challenge yourself first so you can relish in self-satisfaction after. Some examples:

- Pushing through the temptation to get fast food so you might enjoy a healthy, home cooked meal later

- Mustering up a walk and reaching a daily step count goal

- Drinking water instead of soda to lower your blood sugar levels and prevent future medical bills, pain, or prescriptions

Challenges my clients have used to help them control their dopamine response to food include planning and cooking all their dinners at home, spending at least thirty minutes outside in nature, keeping a daily food and mood journal, giving up sugary drinks for a month, and not eating off their kids' plates. Others have gone all out by starting a business, taking evening art or academic classes, joining group fitness classes, or training for big events.

What Motivates You?

It was clear Aniyah was a driven individual who took a lot of pleasure in accomplishing hard things, the most obvious running marathons. Aniyah was motivated **by rewards,** meaning she worked hard because she wanted to gain or accomplish something. For instance, she continuously trained because she enjoyed feeling the runners high, crossing the finish line, and treating herself to a hot shower after a sweat.

Other people are motivated by avoiding **potential consequences**, such as working out to avoid losing strength or feeling weak. The fear of what *could* happen drives these individuals to take action.

It's possible to be motivated by both a reward and avoiding consequences. Table 2.6.6 examines the differences between being driven by reward or avoiding consequences to complete an action.

Action	Driven by Reward	Driven by Avoiding Consequences
Drinking water	To feel hydrated and quench thirst	Prevent dehydration and lightheadedness
Eating at least 24 grams of fiber per day	Regulate digestion	Avoid bloat
Sleeping 7-9 hours	Wake up energized and rested	Reduce under eye circles and falling asleep at the desk
Lifting weights	Build muscle tissue	Decrease risk of osteoporosis

Table 2.6.6

Your Turn

What motivates you to exercise and live healthfully? Is it a reward such as feeling good, or avoiding a consequence such as feeling crummy?

Before we could set up healthy reward-systems, Aniyah and I brainstormed how she could add more food to meet her needs and keep her from overeating at night. We emphasized eating more complex carbohydrates, having plenty of options, and planning meals she actually liked. No more chalky protein bars or fat-free dressing.

Time	Example Meals
Pre-Workout	• A ripe banana with almond butter • Whole food protein bar such as KIND Protein, ZING, or RxBars • Old fashioned oats with cinnamon, dark chocolate chips, and hemp seeds
Post-Workout	• Protein pancakes with freshly ground nut butter as syrup and warm berries • Salmon lox on a seedy bagel with avocado and fruit • Smoothie blended with whey or plant-based protein powder, frozen banana, coconut milk, frozen spinach, and chia seeds
Lunch	• Poke bowl with tuna, avocado, and pickled veggies • Egg salad with sprouted grain bread • Chickpea and farro salad with diced veggies, goat cheese, and Italian dressing • Whole grain flatbread pizza with cheese and onions
Snacks	• Full-fat greek yogurt with apple slices • Energy balls made with oats, dried fruit, peanut butter, and dark cacao nibs • Mixed nuts with a piece of fruit • Cheese stick with grapes • Protein bars made from dates, nuts, and egg whites • Hummus plate with carrots, sliced bell peppers, and flax-seed crackers • Dark chocolate squares with cherries and raspberries
Dinner	• Butternut squash enchiladas • Baked tofu with quinoa, teriyaki, and stir-fry veggies • Turkey meatballs with whole wheat pasta, tomato sauce, and cheese

Table 2.6.7

Unlike diets she had tried in the past, Aniyah was encouraged to eat a variety of foods, including once taboo choices such as chocolate. By prioritizing foods that fueled her sport, she could honor her taste for chocolate without letting her appetite get the best of her.

Your Turn

Review your previous or current meal plans. Using the BNT Protocol and sports nutrition information provided in this chapter, consider how you can modify it to be more substantial. Look for where you can *add* more nutrients via complex carbs, pre-workout fuel, adequate protein, and/or dietary fat.

Old Dog, New Tricks

"To reinforce these new eating patterns, you need to develop a reward system so you still get your dopamine fix," I explained to Aniyah. "Every time you eat a balanced meal or resist the urge to step on the scale, you need to give yourself an immediate reward so your brain learns this is a new behavior to make habitual."

"I feel like a dog. If I do a trick, I get a treat," Aniyah snorted.

She wasn't wrong. Just like teaching a puppy not to pee on a brand new rug from West Elm, Aniyah had to train herself to fuel.

To keep Aniyah focused and excited about making healthy changes, she decided to do 60 days of the **Daily Accountability Program (DAP)**[25]. DAP is a virtual nutrition program where I hold my clients accountable to their health goals with personalized daily messaging, motivation, and encouragement.

"It's like having a dietitian cheerleader in your pocket," I told Aniyah. "Every time you eat, snap a picture or description of your food with either a thumbs up or thumbs down emoji. A thumbs up means

---

[25] *To learn more about The Daily Accountability Program, visit www.orlandodietitian.com/daily-accountability-program*

your meal follows the BNT Protocol. Your goal is to send a thumbs up with eighty percent of your meals."

"It's like a game," Aniyah said. "I want to collect as many thumbs up as possible. I'm already excited for this challenge!"

Other ways reinforce her healthy habits include:

- **A Habit Accountability Partner** such as a friend or trainer.

- **Physical Incentives:** Price out a non-food related reward such as a spa day, weekend trip, or new pair of yoga pants. In a journal or note app, keep track of every healthy habit with a tally mark. Each tally represents a dollar. Once enough tallies have been tracked to pay for the reward, treat yo'self!

- **Habit Trackers:** Use a daily habit tracker to cross off every day you stick to a routine. For instance, drinking 64 ounces of water on Monday, Tuesday, and Thursday earns an X on those dates. As time rolls on, seeing a habit streak is motivating. Digital habit tracking applications include Habitca or Streaks, but a paper copy works great!

- **Sticker Systems:** Remember in kindergarten when you got a sticker or stamp for staying quiet in the hall? It works! Each time you stick to a healthy habit, put a cute sticker on your calendar and watch your streak grow.

- **Mindful Eating Apps:** The Ate App allows users to follow through with healthy eating habits visuals, mindful eating goals, and quick journal prompts.

Your Turn

Which reward systems can you set up to keep you motivated?

"My best friend and running partner is someone who is motivated by avoiding consequences," Aniyah told me. "She trains because she wants to lose weight, sets out to run at sunrise because she doesn't want to wait til it's hot, and stretches religiously to avoid injury. I think she has the same diet issues as me. Any ideas?"

When rewards aren't enough, individuals who are driven to avoid pain should put something on the line to make repeating a desired habit worthwhile. Ideally, the idea of experiencing the consequence should elicit emotional pain or distress.

Ideas to Reinforce Habits with Consequences:

- Daily journaling or meditations reflecting about what negative things happen if you don't change

- Restrict TV, social media, or downtime in the evening until a habit is complete (i.e. *no Netflix unless dinner is cooked*)

- If goals aren't met, commit to paying a certain dollar amount to an undesirable political campaign or sports teams

- Compete with friends or family members to complete actionable goals. Whoever loses has to pay their dues via money, chores, or running dreadful errands

- Delaying a weekend activity until actionable goals are met (i.e. postponing rooftop cocktails or going to the movie theater until the grocery shopping is completed)

"Whether or not you're motivated by rewards or avoiding conse-quences, you should measure your success on your actions and ability to stick to actionable goals, *not* outcomes," I reminded Aniyah, refer-ring to the SMART Goals discussed in Chapter 2. "Instead of treating yourself to a deluxe pedicure when you've lost ten pounds, do it when you've prepped balanced lunches four weeks in a row. Your goal is to reinforce *actionable habits* that lead to the desired result."

Your Turn

Which consequence-avoiding systems can you set up to keep you motivated?

Reclaiming Her Sanity

Before leaving our initial session, Aniyah set the following SMART goals:

1. Eat a carbohydrate-rich pre-workout snack every time she runs

2. Include *at least* one source of complex carbohydrate at every meal and snack to help her energy, recovery, and digestion

3. Replace all artificially-sweetened protein bars with foods made with whole food ingredients such as dates, oats, and nuts

She would reinforce each habit by sending me a picture of her meals with a thumbs up or down emoji for 60 days.

To measure her success, Aniyah would rate her energy, night-time cravings, and endurance on a scale of 1-10. Since she was already tracking her mileage and pace, we'd compare her upcoming workouts with previous months.

Here are some of the messages Aniyah sent to me during our virtual check-ins:

Day 5: *Added sliced banana to my peanut butter toast before my 13-mile run today. I can't remember the last time I ate two carbohydrates at breakfast, but it must be good for me because I beat my average pace! I also rated my energy a 9 when I started and a 7 when I finished, which is much better than my usual 4-5 range.*

Day 11: *Why did I eat three brownies before bed? Because that morning, I saw the scale in my bathroom, stepped on it, and told myself I couldn't eat the brownies. I'm realizing the "I can't have" mindset leads to overeating. I paid the price on my run today when I stopped for my poop loop. Today is a new day, and I'm going to focus on eating foods that fuel me.*

Day 21: *I'm not as obsessed with food. When I get hungry, I go to the fridge and think "What sounds good?" I pick something with complex carbs and protein.*

Day 24: *Today, I ate two energy bars in a row. When I started doing the negative self-talk about how many calories and carbohydrates that was, I stopped and gave myself the freedom to eat both. I noticed I had zero cravings after dinner!*

Day 33: *Yesterday, my son asked for cinnamon rolls. In the past, I would try not to touch them but ultimately give in and eat half the pan after it had been sitting there for an hour or two. This time, I decided to have a cinnamon roll with my eggs and fruit, and I ate it with no guilt at all! I forgot we had leftovers until this morning, and I don't even want one. Crazy!*

Day 44: *No poop loop in over a month! I've never been this regular, and I only feel bloated right before my period. I'm craving chocolate today, so I'm adding dark chocolate chips into my protein pancakes.*

Day 47: *My body really does know how to self-regulate. After taking three days off from running, I was nervous I'd gain weight and wanted to cut carbohydrates. Instead, I ate my usual meals and hit a personal record during today's speed training.*

Day 56: *I am not using the scale and I don't even care how much I weigh anymore. I look and feel better than I have in years, and I am steadily increasing my mileage without hitting any walls. I'm ready for marathon weekend!*

Marathon Weekend

The Dopey Challenge was only two weeks after our 60 days of daily coaching, and Aniyah felt ready for her races. She was consistently meeting her goals to increase carbohydrates and had completely avoided the dreaded Poop Loop.

"I know it's only been a few months, but I can't believe I used to run on empty," Aniyah told me. "I don't think I could have made it this far in my training without you."

"Don't thank me, thank the carbs!" I laughed.

A couple weeks later, I got a text from Aniyah holding up all of her medals with a cheesy grin plastered on her face. Her son was in the photo, posing with one knee on the grass and his hands extended towards Aniyah as if he was presenting her to the world.

Her message read: ...*and now, pancakes!*

I knew she was as proud to finish strong as she was to be a healthy role model for her son.

Shadow Self Integration:

- Fuel an active lifestyle by eating enough total calories and complex carbohydrates.

- Recover from workouts with balanced meals and snacks throughout the day.

- Other than (or along with) weight loss, explore what motivates you to exercise.

- As your increase your food, measure your mood, energy, digestion, and performance levels.

Chapter Takeaways:

- Fueling like an athlete will encourage better eating and lifestyle choices.

- Carbohydrates are the body's preferred source of fuel. Without enough, your energy levels, digestion, and performance suffers.

- The scale is an unreliable way to measure short-term goals due to the many natural shifts in weight that occur throughout the day.

- Foods high protein and fat aid in keeping you full, and should be consumed throughout the day, but are not the best pre-workout fuel.

- Consuming more fiber and water and less sugar alcohols can help with bloat or digestive concerns.

- Endurance athletes benefit from consuming carbs during workouts lasting over 60 minutes.

- Post-workout meals should contain at least 20-40 grams of protein and as many or up to three times the amount of complex carbs.

- To a poorly fueled body, hyperpalatable foods can feel addictive.

- Dieting can feel addicting because the perceived reward from restrictive-behaviors release dopamine, reinforcing the diet-binge cycle.

- Reinforce healthy habits with systems that either reward new behaviors or encourage changing previous behaviors to avoid consequences.

Part 3

Normal Eating for Life

As I hope you've discovered throughout the stories of All-or-Nothing Dieters, there is no "right" way to eat like a normal person. That's up to you (and only you) to decide. Even as you apply the BNT Protocol, I encourage you to modify it based on your experiences, lifestyle, and preferences.

Maybe you'll find you thrive on a plant-based diet, tilting the balance of your eating towards carbohydrates. Or maybe you feel a lot better pushing breakfast until after a morning walk, even if that means eating lunch within two hours instead of three or four. Perhaps you don't feel any different after scarfing greasy tacos than you do after ordering salads, and that's fine, too.

As long as you're making decisions based on your body's needs and don't feel miserable doing it, I'm cheering you on.

Don't forget that as your life evolves, your body and needs will change. This may mean letting go of healthy habits that served you in the past and welcoming new ones that fit your current lifestyle. Moving in with a partner, pregnancy or childbirth, medical diagnoses, exercise routines, and age will impact your version of normal eating, so check in with yourself frequently.

And if you don't achieve the result you want, don't give up on your health or your relationship to food by backsliding into your shadow tendencies with another fad diet. Make subtle adjustments, give your body more time to transform, or work one-on-one with a registered dietitian to identify **sustainable** changes.

No matter how lofty your goals, beginning a diet or medication you cannot stick to for the long haul is **not** worth starting. It's a waste of time, energy, and self-love.

Instead, return to the stories and lessons in this book that resonated with you the most. Reintegrate The BNT Protocol. Remind yourself you **can** see results and improve your health without dieting. After all, there's nothing normal about punishing yourself with food!

Book Club Questions

1. Which of the six sub-archetypes do you most identify with: The Food Tracker, The Perfectionist, The Emotional Eater, The Yo-Yo Dieter, The Binge Eater, or The Cardio Bunny? Do you identify with more than one of the sub-archetypes?

2. Which diets have you been on in your life? How did they work in the short term (1-12 months)? How about in the long term (over 12 months)?

3. How old were you when you went on your first diet?

4. Claire The Food Tracker, Mila The Perfectionist, and Maggie The Yo-Yo Dieter felt a lot of pressure from their primary care-givers to look and eat a certain way. Did you experience this growing up?

5. Who in your life had the biggest impact on your body image? Was it positive or negative?

6. Claire The Food Tracker had signs of **orthorexia**, an eating disorder that involves an unhealthy obsession with healthy or "clean" eating. What orthorexic behaviors have you witnessed that are labeled as healthy but actually disordered (i.e. burning off calories with extra cardio, only buying organic food)?

7. Mila from Chapter 2 learned her people-pleasing was linked to her perfectionism. She believed earning love meant appearing flawless, so she controlled food and obsessed about her weight. If you're a perfectionist, do you associate your diet, health habits, and/or body image with your self-worth? Why?

8. Mila's perfectionism prevented her from being vulnerable, which negatively impacted her relationship to her sister and friends. Share something vulnerable, such as a struggle you've had with food, body image, self-confidence, or dieting.

9. Sarah is an emotional eater who often eats out of frustration, guilt, and depression. If you're An Emotional Eater, which feelings trigger unwanted eating behaviors? What coping tools have you found to help when you are triggered?

10. Refer to the Food Rules worksheet in Chapter 4. Which of these rules have kept you stuck in unhealthy eating patterns and left you feeling deprived, confused, or overwhelmed? Did any rules actually help you, and if yes, how so?

11. The root causes of Josie's binge eating stemmed from her busy and active lifestyle, loneliness, and self-esteem. If you binge or overeat, what are the root causes? What are you doing to address them?

12. Refer to the list of values in Chapter 5. What are your top five values? How are you expressing these values in your life? Do these activities put you into a flow state? When you're in a state of flow, do you think about food?

13. Aniyah The Cardio Bunny thought she was food addict. Do you think it's possible to be addicted to food? Why or why not?

14. How do you plan on integrating the BNT Protocol in your life?

15. Did any of the journal prompts, applicable nutrition tools, or client stories in this book make a lasting impact on you and if so, which ones? Why?

Author Bio

Recovered dieter, registered dietitian nutritionist, Kait Richardson is a wellness junkie (just not in the celery-juice, calorie-counting way). After helping thousands of clients in private practice, she is certain most diet fads, supplements, and weight loss medications are a waste of time, energy, and money. Her mission is to empower women to **quit** yo-yo dieting and start fueling their lives through the power of balanced nutrition and eating whole foods. Her first book, *How to Eat Like a Normal Person*, is a story-workbook inspired by her incredible clients at Nutrition Awareness.

Currently, Kait lives in Orlando, Florida with her fiancé, newborn son, and miniature Aussie, Grits. To work with Kait, visit kaitrichardsonrd.com and follow her on Instagram @kaitrichardsonrd.

Sources

Part 1:

1. Archetypes in Branding: A Toolkit for Creatives and Strategists by Margaret Hartwell (Author), Joshua C. Chen (Author)

2. Mcleod, Saul. "Carl Jung's Theories: Archetypes, Personality, & Collective Unconscious." Simply Psychology, 20 Feb. 2023, https://www.simplypsychology.org/carl-jung.html.

3. Weaver, Tobias. "Embracing the Shadow - Carl Jung." Orion Philosophy, Orion Philosophy, 30 Nov. 2022, https://www.orion-philosophy.com/stoic-blog/the-shadow-carl-jung.

4. Center for Drug Evaluation and Research. "Medications Containing Semaglutide." U.S. Food and Drug Administration, FDA, www.fda.gov/drugs/postmarket-drug-safety-information-patients-and-pro-viders/medications-containing-semaglutide-marketed-type-2-di-abetes-or-weight-loss#:~:text=Are%20there%20concerns%20

with%20compounded,available%20to%20treat%20a%20patient. Accessed 12 Feb. 2024.

5. Wilding JPH, Batterham RL, Davies M, Van Gaal LF, Kandler K, Konakli K, Lingvay I, McGowan BM, Oral TK, Rosenstock J, Wadden TA, Wharton S, Yokote K, Kushner RF; STEP 1 Study Group. Weight regain and cardiometabolic effects after withdrawal of semaglutide: The STEP 1 trial extension. Diabetes Obes Metab. 2022 Aug;24(8):1553-1564. doi: 10.1111/dom.14725. Epub 2022 May 19. PMID: 35441470; PMCID: PMC9542252.

6. Meal Timing and Frequency: Implications for Cardiovascular Disease, www.ahajournals.org/doi/10.1161/CIR.0000000000000476. Accessed 11 May 2023.

7. Metabolic Effects of Intermittent Fasting | Annual Review of Nutrition, www.annualreviews.org/doi/full/10.1146/annurev-nutr-071816-064634. Accessed 11 May 2023.

Part 2:

Chapter 1:

8. Scarff JR. Orthorexia Nervosa: An Obsession With Healthy Eating. Fed Pract. 2017 Jun;34(6):36-39. PMID: 30766283; PMCID: PMC6370446.

9. Avena, Nicole M, et al. "Evidence for Sugar Addiction: Behavioral and Neurochemical Effects of Intermittent, Excessive Sugar Intake." Neuroscience and Biobehavioral Reviews, U.S. National Library of Medicine, 2008, https://www.ncbi.nlm.nih.gov/pmc/articles/PMC2235907/.

10. Kalm, Leah M., and Richard D. Semba. "They Starved so That Others Be Better Fed: Remembering Ancel Keys and the Minnesota Experiment." The Journal of Nutrition, vol. 135, no. 6, 2005, pp. 1347–1352., https://doi. org/10.1093/jn/135.6.1347.

Chapter 3:

11. Weir, K. (2020, April 1). Nurtured by nature. Monitor on Psychology. https://www.apa.org/monitor/2020/04/nurtured-nature

Chapter 4:

12. Ndefo UA, Eaton A, Green MR. Polycystic ovary syndrome: a review of treatment options with a focus on pharmacological approaches. P T. 2013 Jun;38(6):336-55. PMID: 23946629; PMCID: PMC3737989.

13. Nordio M, Basciani S, Camajani E. The 40:1 myo-inositol/D-chiro-inositol plasma ratio is able to restore ovulation in PCOS patients: comparison with other ratios. Eur Rev Med Pharmacol Sci. 2019 Jun;23(12):5512-5521. doi: 10.26355/eurrev_201906_18223. PMID: 31298405.

14. E;, N. M. S. (2019). The 40:1 myo-inositol/d-chiro-inositol plasma ratio is able to restore ovulation in PCOS patients: Comparison with other ratios. European review for medical and pharmacological sciences. https://pubmed.ncbi.nlm.nih.gov/31298405/

15. Jiang, Y., Chen, Y., Wei, L., Zhang, H., Zhang, J., Zhou, X., Zhu, S., Du, Y., Su, R., Fang, C., Ding, W., & Feng, L. (2023b, June 17). DHA supplementation and Pregnancy Complications - Journal of Translational Medicine. BioMed Central. https://translational-medicine.biomedcentral.com/articles/10.1186/s12967-023-04239-8#:~:text=Studies%20suggest%20that%20a%20daily,requirement%20%5B89%2C%20147%5D.

Chapter 5:

13. National Eating Disorders Association: https://www.nationaleatingdisorders.org/

14. Yale University. (2000, November 23). Stress May Cause Excess Abdominal Fat In Otherwise Slender Women, Study Conducted At Yale Shows. ScienceDaily. Retrieved April 24, 2023 from www. sciencedaily.com/releases/2000/11/001120072314.htm

15. Herhaus, B., Ullmann, E., Chrousos, G. et al. High/low cortisol reactivity and food intake in people with obesity and healthy weight. Transl Psychiatry 10, 40 (2020). https://doi.org/10.1038/s41398-020-0729-6

16. Dusheck, J. (2017, May 24). Fitness trackers accurately measure heart rate but not calories burned. News Center. https://med.stanford.edu/news/all-news/2017/05/fitness-trackers-accurately-measure-heart-rate-but-not-calories-burned.html

Chapter 6:

17. Fernández-Elías VE, Ortega JF, Nelson RK, Mora-Rodriguez R. Relationship between muscle water and glycogen recovery after prolonged exercise in the heat in humans. Eur J Appl Physiol. 2015 Sep;115(9):1919-26. doi: 10.1007/s00421-015-3175-z. Epub 2015 Apr 25. PMID: 25911631.

18. Clark, Nancy. Nancy Clark's Sports Nutrition Guidebook. Fifth edition. Champaign, IL, Human Kinetics, 2014.

19. Gearhardt, Ashley & Hebebrand, Johannes. The concept of "food addiction" helps inform the understanding of overeating and obesity: Debate Nonsense. The American Journal of Clinical Nutrition, Volume 113, Issue 2, 274 - 276

20. Yu, Y., Miller, R., & Groth, S.W. (2022, January 28). A literature review of dopamine in binge eating. Retrieved from https://jeatdisord.biomedcentral. com/articles/10.1186/s40337-022-00531-y.

21. Wise, R.A. & Robble, M.A. (2021, January). Dopamine and Addiction. Retrieved from https://www.annualreviews.org/doi/10.1146/annurev-psych- 010418-103337?url_ver=Z39.88-2003&rfr_id=ori%3Arid%3Acrossref. org&rfr_dat=cr_pub++0pubmed.

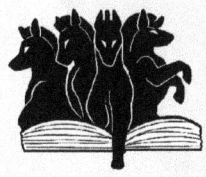

Discover more at
4HorsemenPublications.com

10% off using HORSEMEN10

Printed in the USA
CPSIA information can be obtained
at www.ICGtesting.com
CBHW032049150924
14460CB00001B/2